LICK THE SUGAR HABIT

LICK THE SUGAR HABIT

NANCY APPLETON, PhD

Avery Publishing Group
Garden City Park, New York

Cover Design: William Gonzalez
In-House Editor: Marie Caratozzolo
Typesetter: Bonnie Freid

ISBN 0-89529-695-0 (mass market)

Printed in the United States of America

10 9 8 7 6 5 4 3 2 1

Contents

A Word from the Author,   ix

Acknowledgment,   xi

Foreword,   xiii

Preface,   xv

Introduction,   1

1. I Was a Sugarholic,   3
2. Sugar's Unbalancing Act,   21
3. All About Allergies,   33
4. Destruction of the Immune System,   43
5. The Consequences,   59
6. Sugar's Helpers,   111
7. Stress,   137
8. Sugar, Spice, and Everything Nice,   145
9. A Practical Plan for Attaining and Maintaining Good Health,   153
10. Self-Help Techniques,   173
11. Recipes,   183

Epilogue,   201

Glossary, 203
Notes, 211
Bibliography, 229
Body Chemistry Test Kit Order Form, 241
About the Author, 245
Index, 247

*To all of those
who want to take back control
of their lives
and their health.*

A Word
From the Author

I hope you find the information in this up-to-date edition of *Lick the Sugar Habit* valuable. We eat a tremendous amount of sugar today—an average of 149 pounds per person per year—and more and more people have health problems as a result of this sugar intake, problems for which they are seeking answers.

The basic premise of this book has changed very little from the original. Homeostasis is homeostasis, from the beginning of time to the end of time, and from the beginning of life to the end of life. I have, however, included new research and added valuable new information about sugar that was not known twelve years ago.

The sad truth is that we, as a nation, are eating much more sugar than ever before. This abuse causes a continual insult to our bodies that eventually results in physical problems. Of course, it is not just sugar that causes upset body chemistry. Other things in our twentieth-century lifestyle can also result in a body out of balance, out of homeostasis. The information presented in this book is designed to encourage you to take control of your life and become responsible for maintaining good health through educated choices.

Nancy Appleton, Ph.D.

Acknowledgment

I would like to take this opportunity to recognize a special debt of gratitude to Bruce Pacetti, D.D.S.

His knowledge of the Body Chemistry Principle along with the willingness with which he communicated it to me as well as to others is the bedrock foundation of my successful effort to regain my health. Many of my ideas in this book come from our many talks and his lectures. Not only did I regain my health, but through his understanding and love, a special friendship has developed.

Nancy Appleton, Ph.D.

Foreword

On what do we place the blame for the poor health of modern man? Diet is surely a major factor.

Eggs, that's it. Quick, everyone! Switch to sweet rolls and coffee before the eggs clog your arteries! Oh, no— it's the fat. No more red meat, cut out the butter, watch out for the deadly salad dressing! No, no—salt is the villain. Go for bland, hide the shaker!

Have you noticed that few experts blame sugar? Pure and white, it innocently makes its way into much of our food and into our mouths. If it's so-o-o-o-o-o good, how could it be so bad? Who would not want to believe that it's the omelet rather than the ice cream that's doing us in? Apple pie and ice cream is, after all, the national dish.

Lick the Sugar Habit suggests that sugar eating, our national pastime, is linked to disease, our leading growth industry. We've heard this theory before. Never before, however, has it been presented so clearly and without fanaticism. Nancy Appleton is not saying that sugar is the only cause of disease. She is saying that sugar is a major contributor to the disease process. She presents sugar as one of the stress factors that weaken our defenses against illness.

Sounds reasonable, doesn't it? Eliminating sugar from the diet is also reasonable. Have you ever cut out sugar? That's when life can get very unreasonable. Cold-turkey withdrawal from sugar can bring on the shakes, fever, depression, and headaches. At that point it seems more reasonable to continue the addiction.

Lick the Sugar Habit is a lifesaver, literally. It is a guide to getting unhooked from sugar. Tips on shopping, snacking, supportive friendships, and exercise make this book much more than another synopsis of all the studies on diet and disease.

Even more appealing, Nancy Appleton has been there. Once a sugarholic, she has won the battle against sugar addiction and has been rewarded with vibrant health. The empathy she brings to this subject is genuine. She knows the detrimental effects of sugar.

Are you ready for renewed health and vitality? Will you make the effort to heal and prevent heart disease, cancer, diabetes, arthritis, and osteoporosis?

The most important effort, for many of us, is licking the sugar habit. Unless that is done, all else may be largely wasted effort. The beneficial effects of exercise are lessened by a sugar diet. The roller-coaster emotions of a sugarholic often wreck supportive relationships. A sugar-dependent person is often too tired to function well at home or at work.

If you are ready to be the best that you can be, this book is for you. Sugar-free may be the missing piece in your puzzle for health.

Shirley Lorenzani, Ph.D.

Preface

Nancy Appleton relates her personal story, and with clear scientific analysis gives an understanding of how disease originates and what one can do about it. She also tells how one can improve and monitor one's basic health, and how one can enhance the response to any necessary doctoring.

I have spent the last fifteen years of my professional life doing research, clinically applying and lecturing on an obscure biological principle, which is showing evidence of being the common denominator of all disease. It was like a breath of fresh air for me to see how easily Nancy Appleton understood the Body Chemistry Principle the first time I met and exchanged ideas with her. The Body Chemistry Principle is usually not easily understood by health care practitioners.

The Body Chemistry Principle has to do with the functioning of the body systems that depend upon the body's chemical balances. These systems include the immune system, endocrine system, and digestive system, among others.

Several civilizations have crumbled because of a lack of knowledge about the Body Chemistry Principle. Our civilization is now showing the first signs. Insurance companies are concerned today because statistics show that by 1990, 75 percent of our adult population will have a degenerative disease.

Few Americans today die of old age. Instead, heart attacks, strokes, cancer, and diabetes are the usual causes of death. Arthritis, indigestion, influenza, and constipation are also a normal part of our lives. In the future, will coronary bypasses, artificial hearts and kidneys, hysterectomies, reading glasses, PMS, false teeth, and plastic hip joints also be accepted as normal? They need not be. As always, the fittest will survive and live. The fittest now will be those who understand and somehow apply the Body Chemistry Principle. Appleton's book is a practical introduction to this most vital subject.

Bruce Pacetti, D.D.S.

Introduction

We have heard of the evils of sugar from every writer in the world, except, of course, those from the sugar industry. So what right does Nancy Appleton have to write a book that is going to tell us to stop eating sugar? We've heard that old saw before. But wait, gentle reader! There is something in this book of which you are not aware—good and compelling reasons to avoid the sweet stuff.

The biochemical pathway from ingestion to enzyme function decay is traced in such a clear, understandable way that the most confirmed sugarholic will at least cut down on the intake a smidge. How sugar affects the calcium/phosphorus ratio in the bloodstream, how this seems to be the common pathway of stress, and how this stress can lead to degenerative disease are described and documented. I would get a headache, someone else would get migraine, colitis, asthma, eczema, or depression. A method for self-testing at home and monitoring the nutritional treatment is also presented.

Nancy Appleton's own addiction and recovery give her story a unique viewpoint. She documents the problems stemming from too much sugar and gives self-help techniques and recipes to lick the sugar habit.

A strong case is made for each of us to take responsibility for our own health. Appleton makes it clear that we are responsible for what we eat, think, do, and say. We are not victims of the twentieth-century lifestyle, but many of us do choose a lifestyle that leads to the degenerative disease process.

I recommend this book to everyone who has made personal health a priority, and every person who wants to remove sugar from her or his diet. For sugarholics, *Lick the Sugar Habit* is an absolute must.

Lendon Smith, M.D.

1
I Was a Sugarholic

When I was a child, a bakery truck used to come regularly to the back door of our house. If my mother wasn't around, I could buy anything I wanted and charge it—no one seemed to know who had charged what when the bakery bill came. I would buy six donuts, four nut bars, and a couple of coffee cakes, hide them from the rest of the family, and eat them in private. In two days, all of the goodies would be gone, and I'd wait for the bakery truck and more sweet morsels.

Although I didn't realize it, I was a sugarholic and a chocoholic. Almost from birth I craved the stuff. In my early childhood, I was plagued with bothersome allergies—the signals of an unbalanced body chemistry. My nose ran continually, and so did my eyes. I was constantly sticking fingers in my ears to try to stop the itching, rubbing my fingers over my throat, or even scratching the back of my throat with my tongue for the same reason. Like most people, I misread these body signals and continued my dangerous dietary habits.

My upsetting addiction became worse in my teenage years. I played tennis for four hours a day, every day, and the calories I burned up on the tennis court more than compensated for the calories in the sweets I continued to eat. Therefore, I could consume an incredible amount of sugar and chocolate and not gain weight, even though I was upsetting my body chemistry. After winning a tennis tournament, I would treat myself to two hot-fudge sundaes. When I would lose a tournament, I would eat a whole package of chocolate cookies. Winner or loser, I was a loser. Again, I just wasn't aware of the connection between my sweet addiction, upset body chemistry, and illness.

All I knew at that age was that I wasn't fat—just young, strong, and unhealthy. Every tooth in my mouth was eventually filled with gold or silver. My first bout with pneumonia came at age thirteen, and it put me in the hospital for two weeks. During my second year in college, I had a large tumor removed from my chest, which, after a great deal of expensive investigation, turned out to be a calcium deposit. No one told me that my body was unable to digest milk and calcium properly; no one suggested that the sugar in my diet and other lifestyle factors might be upsetting my body chemistry and causing my increasing health problems. I continued to ignore the signals my body was giving me and, in my ignorance, went right on with my unhealthy lifestyle.

I spent my junior year of college studying in Switzerland, land of chocolate. While in Geneva, I phoned a nearby chocolate factory, explained that I was a food and nutrition major, and asked for a tour. What I really wanted, of course, were the chocolate samples at the end of the line. That little trip fed my habit for about a week. This time, however, the weight game didn't work. Because I was traveling and not playing my usual four hours of tennis every day, I wasn't burning off the excess calories. I came back from Europe thirty pounds overweight, my sugar and chocolate cravings stronger than ever.

My adult life was plagued with boils, canker sores, varicose veins, headaches, constipation, fatigue, colds, flus, and four more bouts with pneumonia—the results of a lifestyle that promoted an upset body chemistry. Each time I became sick with pneumonia, recovery took longer; my immune system was being weakened continually by my dietary habits and my lifestyle. After my last bout with pneumonia, my cough lasted for six months. Every specialist I consulted diagnosed my problem as chronic bronchitis. "Take antibiotics ten days out of the month for the rest of your life," I was told over and over. Not one doctor ever asked, "What do you put in your mouth? What do you eat?"

I was forty years old before I realized how little I knew about nutrition, sugar, allergies, or health. Although I still believed that doctors would take care of me, somehow I just couldn't swallow their diagnoses any easier than I could swallow antibiotics ten days a month for the rest of my life. As my cough continued, I decided to try yoga. I thought that if I stood on my head long enough, the phlegm would come out of my chest. Wrong again. My cough was still there after hours of viewing the world upside down. I hadn't realize that my chemically unbalanced body would produce excess phlegm whether I stood right side up or upside down.

A TWIST OF FATE

A friend suggested that I explore some new ideas on achieving good health by checking out the book section of a health food store. This idea appealed to the book lover in me, and I soon discovered *The Pulse Test*, by Arthur F. Coca, M.D. The author said it was possible to detect food allergies by comparing one's pulse before and after eating the food in question. If my pulse increased ten to twelve beats per minute after I ate the food, Coca suggested, I was not metabolizing that food correctly and was allergic to it.[1]

Being a good do-it-yourselfer, I took my pulse upon awakening and found that I had a resting pulse rate of sixty beats per minute. Remembering that as a child I had suffered from stomach cramps, gas, and allergies after eating ice cream, I drank one glass of milk and took my pulse shortly after. I couldn't believe it—my pulse jumped from sixty beats to eighty in just a few minutes. I repeated the experiment the next morning, with the same results.*

That was eighteen years ago, and it was the beginning of a new life. I began seeing many different types of clinicians: homeopathic doctors, naturopaths, orthomolecular doctors, and clinical ecologists. These doctors deal with a variety of methods for healing the body other than antibiotics and surgery. They changed my diet, gave me supplements, and offered homeopathic medicines that might heal my body. It took me a long time to realize that there is no magic pill and that even a lot of pills together do not make a magic potion. As long as I was feeding my body abusive foods and con-

---

* I must warn you that not all foods to which you've developed allergies alter your pulse. But after ingesting a food, if your pulse rate increases or decreases at least ten beats per minute over the resting rate, the odds are great that you are not metabolizing that food correctly. You have developed an allergic sensitivity to it.

tinually upsetting my body chemistry, all the pills in the world would not help. It's like continuously tapping one's head with a small hammer and wondering why aspirin isn't getting rid of the headache!

Awareness and change take time, and so does healing. There is no such thing as instant health, and the damage I had done to my body over the course of forty years would not be undone overnight. The more I became in touch with my body, the easier it was to discover what it did and didn't need. My body was so out of homeostasis (balance) that it was giving me confusing signals; often the foods that satisfy a craving also deepen the addiction and upset. Getting in touch with my allergies, cravings, addictions, headaches, sneezes, and wheezes was a slow, painful process, but it was also enlightening. Although I often had to backtrack, I eventually learned about my body chemistry and what it took to feel well.

ARE YOU A SUGARHOLIC?

Are you a sugarholic? Is your body giving you any signals? The following quiz will help you determine how pervasive refined sugar is in your lifestyle, and what effect it is having on your body. Refined sugar includes sucrose, honey, fructose, glucose, dextrose, levulose, maltose, raw sugar, turbinado sugar, maple sugar, galactose, brown sugar, dextrine, barley malt, rice syrup, corn sweetener, and corn syrup. All of these are simple sugars. They take very little time to digest and get into the bloodstream, where they perform the same disturbance to your body chemistry as table sugar. These substances are found in donuts, processed foods, jams and jellies, ice cream, candy bars, packaged cereals, soft drinks, ketchup, beer, chewing tobacco, chewing gum, and any product that lists sugar among its ingredients.

Answer each of the following questions as truthfully as you can; you're not going to be graded, and no one is looking over your shoulder. Be honest with yourself—your health depends on it.

	True	False
1. I do not eat refined sugar every day.		
2. I can go for more than a day without eating some type of sugar-containing food.		
3. I never have cravings for sugar, coffee, chocolate, peanut butter, or alcohol.		
4. I've never hidden candy or other sweets around my home in order to find and eat them later.		
5. I can stop after eating one piece of candy or one bite of pastry.		
6. There are times when I have no sugar of any kind in my home.		
7. I can go for three or more hours without eating and not experience the shakes, fatigue, perspiration, irritability, depression, or anxiety.		
8. I can have candy and other sweets in my home and not eat them.		
9. I do not eat something sweet after every meal.		

	True	False
10. I rarely drink coffee and eat donuts or sweet rolls for breakfast.	____	____
11. I can go for more than an hour after waking up in the morning without eating.	____	____
12. I can go from one day to the next without drinking a sweetened soft drink.	____	____

If you answered "false" to more than four of these statements, chances are you are sugar-sensitive. You are probably allergic to sugar and also addicted to it—the same way an alcoholic is addicted to alcohol. You crave sugar, have withdrawal symptoms when you don't get it, and probably feel better for a short time after you've eaten it. In eating sugar to feel better, you are actually making your condition worse.

If you answered "false" to four statements or fewer, it doesn't necessarily mean you don't have a problem with sugar. You may not be addicted to it, but perhaps you don't quite realize just how much sugar you're eating.

How much sugar does the average American consume? This question is more difficult than it seems. Until the 1970s, most of the sugar we ate came from sugar beets and sugar cane and was called sucrose. Then in the '70s, sugar from corn—corn syrup, fructose, dextrose, dextrine, and/or high fructose corn syrup (HFCS)—began to gain popularity as a sweetener because it was much less expensive than the sugar produced from beets or cane. In order to determine an accurate amount of sweeteners that the average person consumes, it is necessary to combine sucrose and corn sweeteners. Unfortunately, when those in the sugar industry or others with a vested interest in sugar write about sugar consumption, they do not include corn sweeteners. This is deceiving. Many publications have claimed that we are eating less sugar today than we were ten years ago. While it is true that we are eating less sugar, we are consuming a lot more corn sweeteners.

During the 1980s, sugar consumption dropped 33 percent, and corn sweetener consumption averaged 39.6 pounds per person. By 1994, the corn sweetener rate doubled to 83.2 pounds per person. According to the USDA's *Sugar and Sweeteners*, a quarterly newsletter, the total consumption of these two major sweeteners, which include sucrose, HFCS, glucose, dextrose, honey, maple syrup, and other edible syrups, increased from 124.4 pounds per person in 1980, to 149.2 pounds per person in 1994.[2]

One of the problems with regulating sugar consumption is being able to identify the foods that contain it. It's not always obvious. Many foods, however, do contain sugar. For example, you may be surprised to learn that:

• Many meat packers feed sugar to animals prior to slaughter. This improves the flavor and color of cured meat.

• Sugar (in the form of corn syrup and dehydrated molasses) is often added to hamburgers sold in restaurants to reduce shrinkage.

• The breading on many prepared foods contains sugar.

• Before salmon is canned, it is often glazed with a sugar solution.

• Some fast-food restaurants sell poultry that has been injected with a flavorful honey solution.

• Sugar is used in the processing of luncheon meats, bacon, and canned meats.

• Sugar is found in such unlikely items as bouillon cubes and dry-roasted nuts.

• Sugar is found in beer, wine, and other alcoholic beverages. Champagne and cordials have an unusually high sugar content.

• Sugar is often added to the syrup in canned fruits.

• Peanut butter and many dry cereals (even corn flakes) contain sugar.

• Some salt contains sugar.

• Almost half the calories found in most commercial ketchups come from sugar.

• Over 90 percent of the calories found in the average can of cranberry sauce come from sugar.

It is important to be aware (and beware) of the sugar-laden world around you. Remember, according to statistics, the average person eats over 10 pounds of sugar each month, nearly 4½ cups per week or 30 to 33 teaspoonfuls every day. That's over 20 percent of our daily caloric intake spent on a refined food that upsets body chemistry and has no nutritional value. Refined sugar is 99.4 to 99.7 percent pure calories—no vitamins, minerals, or proteins, just simple carbohydrates.[3]

HOW YOU FEEL IS UP TO YOU

My experience is a classic example of what I call the "degenerative disease process." All of my ailments were caused by the substances I put into my body. The excess sugar that I ate so obsessively led to a measurable disturbance of the mineral relationships in my system. This mineral imbalance made my digestive enzymes incapable of digesting food properly. I developed classic allergic symptoms due to the toxicity and the undigested food, which was wearing out my immune system.[4] Eventually, this mineral imbalance caused the buildup of a severe nonfunctioning calcium excess in my chest. My strong but upset and toxic body manifested one continuous disease process. This process, which started with the excess consumption of sugar, ended in tooth decay, pneumonia, bronchitis, and a variety of other ailments. It was only after I removed the sugar from my diet that my body was able to regain health. I realized for the first time that if I stopped doing to my body what I had done to make it sick, my body would heal itself.

Having shared my health saga with many people, I know now that many of us go through life not knowing what it is to feel well. We are somewhere between health and the disease process most of the time, our symptoms and body signals of toxicity oscillating between not-so-bad and miserable. Since that is all we know, we start believing this is how everyone feels.

Still, it is possible to feel better—and if you really want to, chances are that you can. *It is up to you.* You can either choose to make yourself sick by ingesting harmful substances, or you can listen to your body's signals and do what it requires to heal itself.

If you choose to ignore the signals of upset and toxicity that your body is sending, you will force doctors to use stronger and more dangerous techniques, and relegate yourself to the role of victim. Doctors are accustomed to treating conditions that have progressed to a point at which there are serious complaints (severe pain, heart palpitations, swollen joints, or rapid weight loss).

They see these drastic conditions and they take drastic measures.

SUGAR—THE SOUR FACTS

Now, I don't eat any sugar, and I know many others who don't, so many of you must be getting more than the 149 pounds that the average person consumes in a year. Your body needs only two teaspoons of blood sugar at any time in order to function properly. This amount can be obtained easily through the digestion of unrefined carbohydrates, protein, and fats. Even if we ate no glucose or refined sugar at all, our bodies would still have plenty of blood sugar. Every extra teaspoon of refined sugar you eat works to throw your body out of balance and compromise its health.

Ironically, the initial damage done by excess refined sugar makes it that much harder to give up the sweet stuff. Refined sugar is made up of two simple sugars, glucose and fructose. When a person eats sugar continually, the body becomes inefficient at manufacturing glucose from complex carbohydrates, protein, and fats. The mechanisms in the body that perform this task shut down from disuse, causing the blood glucose level to drop. The cravings, perspiration bouts, shakes, and depression that commonly follow send the sugarholic running for the nearest candy bar or cookie jar, and the vicious cycle continues. These sweets may bring the blood sugar back to normal for the moment, but the body chemistry is still being upset. When the individual gets to the point at which his or her body chemistry cannot rebalance, health breakdowns result.

Refined sugar, as tempting as it may be in all those cakes, candies, and cups of coffee, is, in fact, more of a

Sugar-Coating
the Truth

*Abraham Lincoln once said, "You can fool all of the people
some of the time, and some of the people all of the time, but
you can't fool all of the people all of the time." Obviously
Lincoln hadn't been trying to get information about sugar
from the government.*

*In 1977, the United States Senate's Select Committee
on Nutrition and Human Needs issued a report entitled
"Dietary Goals for the United States." The report was
highly critical of "America's eating patterns," which, it
declared, "represent as critical a public health concern as
any now before us."[1] Forcefully, the Committee related the
American people's excess sugar consumption with tooth
decay, diabetes, obesity, and heart disease and called for a
40 percent reduction in sugar intake. The senate never
issued another report on nutrition. And this 1977 report is
hard to come by—negotiated out of print.*

*In 1986, the Food and Drug Administration (FDA) issued
a report on American sugar consumption and its possible ill
effects on health. The conclusions in this report were based
largely on information that had been published in medical
journals, not on the FDA's own scientific research. One conclusion indicated that the consumption of sugar in large
quantities—anywhere from 25 to 50 percent or more of one's
caloric intake—could result in one or more of the the following
complications: diabetes mellitus, glucose intolerance, hypoglycemia, hyperglycemia, cardiovascular risks, behavioral*

changes, excess calcium secretion in the urine, gallstones, and mineral deficiencies. However, the report went on to say that Americans need not worry about such medical problems (with the exception of tooth decay) because sugar consumption in this country is not that high.[2]

The report further stated that the figure of 124 pounds of sugar, which was believed to be consumed by the average American in 1985, actually indicated the amount of sugar manufactured in the United States in 1985, not consumed. According to the report, the average American ate only 40 pounds of sugar per year (about 8 to 12 teaspoons a day). So what happened to the extra 84 pounds of sugar that was allegedly manufactured but not eaten? Supposedly, some of it was used in pet food, some was exported or stored, and some if it was lost during shipping and processing.

Unable to take the FDA's word for it, I started doing my own research. Shortly after the report came out, I telephoned the FDA and spoke to Dr. Hiltje Irausquin, one of the authors of the report. When asked how she and the other researchers arrived at the figure of 40 pounds of sugar as the average person's intake per year, she admitted the FDA's method was neither scientific nor sound. Conclusions were based on a questionnaire that had been sent to 5,000 people who had kept a weekly diet diary. Dr. Irausquin assured me that in the future, a better method would have to be used.

Still unconvinced that the average American consumed only 40 pounds of sugar per year, I phoned the Soft Drink Association. I spoke with Irene Melvin, who sent me a report entitled "Estimated Annual Production and Consumption of Soft Drinks." The report showed that in 1985, the average person in the United States drank the equivalent of approximately 486 12-ounce cans of soft drinks, 100 of which were sugar-free.[3] *Each sugary soft drink contains approximately 10 teaspoons of sugar. Multiplying that 10 teaspoons by the 386 cans of sugared soft drinks consumed that year, meant that the per capita consumption of sugar from soft drinks alone was 11 teaspoons per day. So if we believe the FDA's claim that the average American consumed 40 pounds of sugar in 1985 (12 teaspoons per day), then we must also believe that only 1 teaspoon per day came from items other than soft drinks. Hardly believable when you think of all the cookies, candies, cakes, ice creams, jams, jellies, fruit yogurts, and other sugary foods we eat!*

I believe the FDA made a gross error. Other sources I have read state that the average American consumed more than 120 pounds of sugar in 1985. The University of California's **Berkeley Wellness Letter** *estimated a whopping 133 pounds per year, accounting for 20 to 25 percent of all calories, and 500 to 600 calories per person per day in 1985!*[4]

As I mentioned earlier, recent government research shows that in 1994, sugar consumption averaged 149 pounds per person per year. Yet the government doesn't seem concerned; and the seemingly vague position it currently holds regarding sugar makes it difficult for the American public to obtain accurate information. It seems the less we know about how much sugar is contained in our diets, the less we have to worry about. With the skyrocketing costs of health care and the increasing incidents of degenerative conditions, we all have a lot to worry about.

pharmaceutical drug than it is a nurturing food. The minerals needed to digest sugar—chromium, manganese, cobalt, copper, zinc, and magnesium—have been stripped from the sugar during the refining process.

This, in turn, forces the body to deplete its own mineral reserves to process the sugar.

Glucose, as high in calories as refined sugar, is actually a predigested food that undergoes no processing at all in the stomach or intestines. Yet there is no law requiring that glucose be listed with other ingredients on the label of any package! And the food industry commonly uses glucose as a cheap filler. Since glucose is not as sweet as sugar and, therefore, unrecognizable, many people consume large quantities of it unknowingly. If you eat foods such as packaged cereals, commercial baked goods, and processed meats, chances are you're getting more hidden refined sugars than you bargained for—maybe 149 pounds more per year!

This high sugar consumption hasn't always been the case. It is only in the last two centuries that sugar has become a staple of the American diet. In colonial America, table sugar cost $2.40 a pound, as compared to today's cost of $.35 a pound. Sugar was an expensive luxury then, and a cube of sugar in a Christmas stocking was considered a real treat. In 1795, a large-scale method of granulating sugar was devised, and Louisiana farmers began growing sugar cane as a major crop. Sugar prices went down, availability went up, and Americans began eating too much of it.

The history of sugar consumption was easy to document until the 1970s. Virtually all of our sweeteners came from sugar beets or sugar cane until that time; and they were called sugar or sucrose. After that time, high fructose corn syrup (HFCS) was introduced, first in the United States, then in Japan, and then to the rest of the world. In the United States, more than 50 percent of our processed sugar comes from HFCS. For clarification in this book, the term "sugar" refers to all sugars that come from cane, beets, and corn.

Human evolution has not yet caught up with the sugar industry. For many thousands of years, mankind ate no refined sugar at all. Early man ate meat, some vegetables, fruit, seeds, and nuts. The past two hundred years of sugar is merely a moment compared to this, and our bodies have not yet evolved mechanisms to cope with this glut. Therefore, our bodies are not able to metabolize large amounts of sugar on a daily basis. In compensating for the excess, our glands and organs become overworked and exhaused, and eventually they malfunction. This scenario is an initiator of the degenerative disease process.

LISTEN TO YOUR BODY

If you're a sugarholic, as I was, your body is telling you quite bluntly that sugar is causing problems. Addiction is closely related to allergy; the body has become so accustomed to compensating for the presence of the allergenic substance that when the substance is removed, withdrawal symptoms occur. Your sugar cravings are a direct indication that sugar is at work destroying your body.

There are many other ways in which a sugar problem can manifest itself. You may become allergic to other foods (see Chapter 3). You may experience headaches, joint pains, gas pains, bloating, fatigue, and other ailments that are not easily traced to sugar. For this reason, many who are not necessarily sugarholics, who do not feel cravings for sugar or a need to indulge their sweet tooth, refuse to believe that sugar could be the cause of such physical problems. They continue their dietary indiscretions, and their disease process is allowed to advance.

Therefore, it's important to understand exactly how sugar, even a little sugar, starts this chain reaction. The pages that follow represent a step-by-step journey down this pathway to degenerative disease. You'll learn how refined sugars throw the body out of balance and can cause food allergies, endocrine problems, hypoglycemia, diabetes, tooth decay, osteoporosis, arthritis, cancer, and many other degenerative diseases. You'll discover concrete self-help techniques to help rid yourself of these problems. Following these techniques can lead you to a philosophy of responsibility instead of one of helplessness in health matters.

When you realize that you have created your own ill health, you can also discover the good news—that through some simple lifestyle changes, you can be responsible for bringing yourself back to good health.

2
Sugar's Unbalancing Act

Minerals are essential to many bodily functions. They give rigidity to the hard tissues of the body: the bones and teeth. They also help to maintain a balance in the blood and body tissues between acidity and alkalinity. Some minerals have specific functions in the transmission of nerve impulses throughout the body, others are important in the process of digestion.

Those minerals that are highly essential to the body include: *calcium* and *phosphorus*, which, in addition to building strong bones, activate enzymes needed for important metabolic functions; *magnesium*, which is both a structural material and an enzyme catalyst; *iron*, which contributes to enzymes and is an important part of the blood's hemoglobin; *iodine*, which is necessary to the proper functioning of the thyroid gland; and *zinc*, without which the enzyme alcohol dehydrogenase cannot perform its function of oxidizing alcohol in the liver.[1]

The average person consumes 20 to 25 percent of his or her calories from some form of refined sugar. Many people think that they can eat anything they want as long as they take their multivitamin and mineral pill daily. Sugar so upsets the body chemistry that it doesn't matter what else you put in your mouth; neither healthful food nor junk food will digest properly.

Somewhere along the path of creating health for myself, I realized how important it was to have enough of the right vitamins, minerals, essential fatty acids, and amino acids in my diet. I would regularly sit down to a nutrient-filled meal, then, because I had eaten such healthy food, I would treat myself to a piece of chocolate cake or other sugar-laden dessert—negating many positive effects the nutrients might have had.

As long as refined sugars are eaten, many essential nutrients will be unavailable to the body. The recommended daily allowance (RDA) of vitamins and minerals set by the U.S. government is not a valid measure for health. Even if people do meet daily requirements through food or supplements, if they also eat sugar, the sugar will change their body chemistry, and the cells will not be able to fully benefit from those vitamins and minerals. The nutrients may actually become toxic to the body.

RESEARCH

The disastrous effect of sugar on the calcium-phosphorus ratio was first discovered by Dr. Melvin Page, a dentist. Dr. Page noted bone loss in his patients, and at first believed this to be the result of a calcium deficiency. However, these patients all showed normal calcium levels in their blood. Page consulted several physicians inquiring how this could be, and the answer was always the same: "If there are eight to ten units of calcium in the blood, then there is enough calcium in the body." What these physicians didn't realize—and many still don't— is that minerals work only in relation to each other.

Fortunately Page did not accept their explanation. He started looking at other minerals in the body. He found that if he could get a patient's calcium-phosphorus ratio to be the optimum 10 to 4, the symptoms that led to tooth decay and bone loss, as well as many other negative symptoms, would simply go away. Through further investigation, he discovered that sugar caused the phosphorus and calcium levels to either decrease or increase. When the calcium level increased, the phosphorous level decreased. And when the calcium decreased, the phosphorus increased. Excess calcium was unable to be used optimally because it was not in correct balance with phosphorus. Once Dr. Page took his patients off sugar and put them on a diet of whole foods, their dental problems began to disappear as did many other problems.[2]

Researchers have found that ingesting sugar increases the rate at which we excrete calcium.[3] If, when we eat sugar, our blood calcium increases and we also excrete it, we must be pulling the calcium from our bones and tissues, where it is stored. Calcium depletion of the bones makes them fragile and leads to osteoporosis. Often a doctor will recommend taking extra calcium to combat this depletion. However, supplemental calcium can become toxic if it is not in proper balance with the body's other minerals. It would be far better to first cut sugar out of the diet; sugar is one of the main substances that throws the body chemistry out of balance—out of homeostasis—and causes calcium deficiency in the first place.

Homeostasis is the wonderful balance in the body. It involves a continual fine-tuning of the body chemistry.

A relatively stable state of equilibrium or a tendency between elements

The vitamins and minerals in our body chemistry are always fluctuating a little. This is normal. However, when the fluctuations become too great for too long, disease creeps in. When our body is in homeostasis, the glands secrete the correct amount of hormones into the bloodstream and the body systems function optimally. These functions include, among others, the regulation of mineral ratios, the production of enzymes, and the total digestive process, which permits and encourages the proper performance of the internal functions that are necessary for growth, healing, and life itself. Good health requires the proper functioning of all of these controls. When the body is in homeostasis it is healing. When it is out of homeostasis, through life's indiscretions, it is on the degenerative disease path. Disease is that simple.

Disease may begin in a single organ or system, but the interdependence and close coordination of the many bodily functions, which cooperate so beautifully in health, may be upset by a chain reaction when one breaks down.[4] This is the meaning of holistic health, the entire body is involved in both health and disease.

Sugar (even as little as two teaspoons) can cause the body's micronutrients to change radically, throwing the blood chemistry out of homeostasis. Some minerals increase, some decrease, and delicate ratios are disturbed. In healthy people the minerals come back into relationship soon; in sick people the minerals stay out of proper relationship for hours, and sometimes the balance does not return at all. When minerals are out of balance day after day, year after year, and possibly through generations, the body's ability to balance back into homeostasis is exhausted. The body can no longer fine-tune itself.

MINERAL RELATIONSHIPS

In the body, minerals rule over all other nutrients. Vitamins, proteins, enzymes, and amino acids, as well as fats and carbohydrates require minerals for activity. Trace minerals, such as zinc, chromium, and copper, are needed in small amounts. They are, however, no less important to the functioning of the body than are the macro minerals—calcium, magnesium, potassium, sulphur, and chloride—which are needed in larger amounts. There are eighty-four known minerals, seventeen of which are considered to be essential in human nutrition. If there is a shortage of just one of these essential minerals, the balance of activity in the entire system can be thrown off. Deficiency of a single mineral can negatively impact the entire chain of life, rendering other nutrients ineffective and useless.[5]

As shown in the mineral wheel in Figure 2.1, minerals work only in relation to one another. If the body is deficient in one mineral, most other minerals won't function as well. Conversely, when one mineral increases and another does not, the mineral that has increased may become toxic because it is no longer in correct ratio or relationship with the other one. That is why some vitamins and minerals are prescribed only in conjunction with certain others.[6] It's like trying to make French toast with a whole loaf of bread and only one egg; you may have the right ingredients, but you won't get French toast.

This interrelationship of minerals, and the damage that can be caused by disturbing it, is readily seen in the case of calcium and phosphorus (as discussed in Dr. Page's work on page 22), two of the most important minerals in the body. The normal ratio of these minerals is 10 units of calcium to 4 units of phosphorus, or 2.5

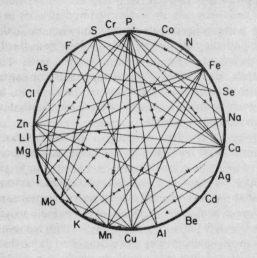

Figure 2.1 Mineral-Relationship Wheel
As this wheel shows, each mineral depends on other minerals to function properly.

Dr. Paul Eck, Analytical Research Labs, Phoenix, Arizona.

times as much calcium as phosphorus. Since minerals work properly only when they are in the correct ratio, if the phosphorus decreases, the functioning calcium also decreases. If there are only 2 units of phosphorus, then only 2.5 times that, or 5 units of calcium, will be functioning; the rest of the calcium can become harmful. On the other hand, if calcium increases to a level of 12 units, but the phosphorus level remains at 4, then the extra 2 units of calcium can become toxic.

If only 5 units of calcium are functioning, then the body is getting only half of the calcium it needs, since the optimum amount is 10. Therefore, it is possible to have both toxic calcium and a calcium deficiency in the body at the same time, a seeming contradiction. Toxic or nonfunctioning calcium can cause kidney stones, arthritis, hardening of the arteries, gallstones, bone spurs, cataracts, and tooth plaque. In my case, toxic calcium had been accumulating in my body since birth, and eventually resulted in a large calcium deposit that was removed from my chest.

Many studies have confirmed the importance of proper mineral relationships. For instance, in response to epidemiological research that indicated a large portion of populations in industrialized countries consume less than the recommended amounts of magnesium, a study was performed in which rats were fed a magnesium-deficient (200 milligrams a day) diet for ten weeks. This low-magnesium diet caused impaired tissue distribution of zinc. Not only was there a reduction in blood zinc, there was an above-normal zinc increase in the intestines and kidneys.[7] I believe if other minerals had been tested during this study, they would have also shown an increase or decrease.

deals with distribution of and control of disease in population

THE ENDOCRINE SYSTEM

Your body's endocrine system determines which minerals are going to be the most affected by sugar. This system, which is made of several organs called glands, is the automatic pilot of the processes in the body. It regulates all involuntary or unconscious activities. Respiration; heartbeat; digestion, assimilation, and elimination of food; body temperature; physical integrity; equilibrium; and balanced body chemistry all come under the supervision of one or more of the endocrine glands.

The endocrine glands include the pituitary, the thyroid, the parathyroid, the hypothalamus, the adrenals, part of the pancreas, the thymus, the pineal, and the gonads. All of these glands are characterized by their ability to produce chemical messengers called hormones, which are secreted directly into the bloodstream and determine how the body works. The intake of harmful foods like sugar can reduce the efficiency of some glands, causing a decrease or increase in hormone secretion, or an altered hormonal composition. This, in turn, can have a detrimental effect on the body chemistry.

Each of us has inherited some weak glands and some strong glands. If our body stays in balance because of a healthy lifestyle, neither the weak nor the strong glands will hurt us. However, if we destroy our body chemistry through dietary indiscretions, our weak glands will become exhausted and our strong glands, in compensating for the weak ones, will become exhausted as well.

The endocrine system is designed so that many glands have an opposite in terms of these strengths and weaknesses.[8] Examples of corresponding glands are indicated in Figure 2.2.

If you have a genetic potential to be, say, a 6 out of a possible 10 rating in the thyroid, then the pancreas will be a 10. When your body chemistry becomes unbalanced, the pancreas may overcompensate and go up to a 12. Since the function of the pancreas is to secrete insulin, sodium bicarbonate, and pancreatic enzymes, an excess of these substances may occur. If you were also born with a weak anterior pituitary, the pancreas would have to work even harder to compensate.

Each person's inherited endocrine system produces individual psychological and physical characteristics. A person with an overactive thyroid, whose body chemis-

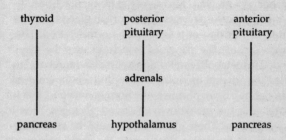

Figure 2.2 . Corresponding Glands in the Endocrine System

try is routinely upset, will suffer with bouts of heavy perspiration, emotional ups and downs, and hyperactivity. People with a weak postpituitary tend to become extremely emotional. If they go to a sad movie and their body chemistries are in balance, they will likely cry. If they go to a sad movie, and upset their body chemistries by eating candy and drinking soft drinks, they will likely become devastated, even hysterical.

This was the case with me. I was born with a potential toward a weak postpituitary and anterior pituitary in addition to a weak thyroid. I remember many a time going to a movie as a child and crying my heart out. Everyone around me thought I was crazy. I can vividly remember seeing a movie called *No Sad Songs for Me*. It was about a mother of two young children who was dying of cancer. She maneuvered her husband to fall in love with his secretary so he would have someone to love him and their children after she died. I cried through half the movie, all the way home, and I even cried myself to sleep. Of course, the sugar I was eating so obsessively had thrown my body chemistry out of balance, which was causing my extreme reactions.

When a person ingests sugar, certain glands are accelerated to function at a faster-than-normal speed. These glands include the pancreas, which secretes the insulin needed to metabolize sugar, and a part of the adrenal gland called the adrenal medulla, which produces epinephrine (adrenaline). Epinephrine is the hormone responsible for stimulating the breakdown of stored glycogen back to usable glucose. These glands also control the assimilation of calcium; the faster they work, the more calcium is absorbed into the blood, resulting in the calcium-phosphorus imbalance discussed earlier.

Other glands, such as the thyroid and the adrenals, are reduced to a slower-than-normal activity level due to sugar. These are the glands that control the assimilation of phosphorus. Just as the overstimulation of the calcium regulators causes an increase in calcium, the suppression of these phosphorus regulators leads to a decrease in phosphorus. Such a decrease, as we have seen, means a decrease in usable calcium, even as the overall calcium level in the blood rises. The vicious cycle continues.

The levels of calcium and phosphorus in the blood indicate whether the endocrine system is in balance or not. Since the endocrines are those glands that regulate metabolism, it is obvious that their balance or lack of balance will result in the health or lack of health in an individual.

ENZYMES

Metabolism is the process by which food is broken down into essential nutrients that can be absorbed by the cells of the body. This function is performed by enzymes, and enzymes are influenced by minerals—minerals that sugar works to unbalance. Most enzymes are mineral-dependent. Minerals work along with enzymes not only to digest food but also to bring about certain necessary biochemical functions in the body. Chymotrypsin, for example, is a zinc-dependent enzyme needed to fine-tune carbohydrate metabolism; it is also used to counteract inflammation and reduce swelling.[9]

Every food we eat needs to be digested and metabolized by a variety of enzymes before it can be used by our cells. Enzymes will work without the proper functioning minerals to help them out. If the usable minerals in the body decrease, as in the presence of sugar, they will not be able to aid in proper enzyme functions. When we ingest sugar, it is difficult for the body to digest anything in the small intestine because of the lack (or decrease) of functioning enzymes. Therefore, when you eat sugar, any food that is in the stomach at the time will become the food to which you can become allergic. This continued inability to digest a particular food eventually results in an allergy to that undigested, decomposing food. How this occurs is described in the next chapter.

3
All About Allergies

The word *allergy* carries with it a vision of sneezes, weepy eyes, and runny noses. Of course, allergic reactions are more extensive than these. Research shows that many allergies are caused by food that is not properly digested. As discussed in Chapter 2, undigested food is often due to unbalanced mineral relationships, which prevent digestive enzymes from functioning properly. Nutrients in partially digested or undigested food cannot be made available to the body, and this lack of nutrients compromises the body's ability to function optimally.

When these undigested food microparticles enter the bloodstream they can travel to different parts of the body and play havoc. If the particles go to the head, the result can be a headache, fatigue, or dizziness; in other parts of the body, the microparticles can cause joint pain or swelling, often in the ankles, legs, or hands.

FOOD ALLERGIES

Not coincidentally, the foods to which most people are allergic—milk, corn, wheat, and chocolate—are those foods most commonly eaten with sugar. Sugar is added to milk to make ice cream; wheat is blended with sugar in a tempting variety of cookies and cakes; corn in the form of corn sweetener is used to sweeten most processed foods; and chocolate is impossible to eat without the addition of some sugar. It is primarily because we eat these foods so often and in large quantities that we are more than likely to become allergic to them.

Eggs also commonly cause allergic reactions. I am convinced that this is because eggs are commonly eaten at breakfast along with sugary foods (donuts, toast with jelly, Danish) and sweet fruit juices. A ten-ounce glass of orange juice contains the juice of approximately six to eight large oranges—the equivalent of nine teaspoons of sugar. Some people regularly eat a breakfast that includes eggs and orange juice. The simple sugar from the orange juice can exhaust the enzymes needed for proper digestion of the eggs. Thus, the body can develop an allergy to eggs.

You may find it hard to believe that orange juice, with all of that vitamin C, could do anything bad to the body. In order to prove the theory that the sugar in orange juice can cause a mineral imbalance, I conducted an experiment. I wanted to see what would happen to the body's calcium-phosphorus ratio during the four-hour period after orange juice had been ingested. I gave ten ounces of orange juice to two healthy people. Using the Body Chemistry Test (see page 161), I discovered that the orange juice altered their calcium-phosphorus ratio just as plain table sugar did. There is enough simple sugar in ten ounces of orange juice to change the body's mineral relationships, making the juice just as harmful as cookies and coffee cake.

If you are one who often enjoys a breakfast that includes eggs and juice, have the juice when you first wake up. Then get dressed before eating the rest of your breakfast. This will give the juice time to get through your stomach; when the eggs get there, the hydrochloric acid and pepsin in the stomach will be able to digest the protein without the interference of the sugar from the orange juice. You might also choose to limit the amount of juice you drink or try diluting the juice with water. Better still, eat the whole fruit instead. When you eat an orange or an apple, your digestive process is slowed due to the fruit's fiber. Because digestion takes longer, the fruit's sugar is secreted into the bloodstream slowly, not quickly as it is in its juice form. In addition, the fiber works to keep the intestinal tract clean and help prevent constipation.

Over thirty years ago, Dr. Theron Randolph, a researcher, learned that people who were allergic to corn reacted more acutely to cornmeal when corn sugar was added than when the cornmeal was eaten alone. The conclusion drawn was that these people were more allergic to sugar than they were to corn. What the researcher didn't realize was that the added corn sugar could have caused an allergic reaction to any food the subjects ate.[1] Sugar, and this includes corn sugar, depletes enzymes. When there is a deficiency of enzymes, it is possible to become allergic to any undigested food that is sitting in the stomach and intestines.

Once a person's body chemistry is unbalanced, any number of life experiences can trigger an allergic response. In fact, our susceptibility to allergies begins at

birth. If a mother has nutritional and enzymatic deficiencies, and therefore an unbalanced body chemistry,
the body chemistry of her infant may also be unbalanced.[2]

Dr. George Ulett tested blood from the umbilical
cords of a number of newborns before any food had
entered their gastrointestinal tracts. Through these tests,
he found that some of the babies showed a sensitivity to
foods to which one or both of the parents were allergic.
These sensitivities set the stage for the child to have
allergic reactions later in life. Dr. Ulett felt that in some
instances only the allergic tendency was inherited; specific food allergies were acquired through exposure.
Any food was a potential allergen.[3]

When I was a baby, I threw up my milk every morning. Worried, my mother asked my doctor what to do.
The doctor advised her to let me sleep in the vomit—that
this would cure me. Well, it did cure me of vomiting, but
it did not cure my body's violent reaction to milk. I was
still allergic to the milk, but I didn't like sleeping in the
vomit, so my body adapted and I stopped throwing up.
However, my body reacted in a different way. I developed a large calcium deposit in my chest, which had to
be removed when I was in college. The calcium from the
milk caused the deposit, which had started growing
when I was a baby. The moral of the story is that I should
have listened to my body. The stuffy nose and watery
eyes that plagued me as I was growing up were signals
of undigested protein, of my body's reaction to a food
that was not being digested. Our bodies are constantly
telling us things—things we are often unwilling to hear.

If a baby is born with an unbalanced body chemistry,
future years may bring on many problems. Dr. Joel
Wallach reported a case in which a child developed a

rash twelve hours after the nursing mother ate straw-
berry pie. When the mother stopped eating the pie, the
rash went away. When the mother went back to the pie,
the infant's rash came back. In Sweden, colic in babies
was found to occur when the infants' mothers drank
milk. It was confirmed immunologically that the breast
milk contained cow's milk antigen. In Japan, the eating
of eggs by a nursing mother coincided with the development of eczema in her child.[4]

When a baby is born prematurely and has an unde-
veloped digestive, immune, or endocrine system, that
baby will have difficulty digesting foods. Breastfeeding
a child for the first six months is the best way to help
encourage healthy systems. This is especially important
for an allergic baby or one that comes from an allergic
family.

Another way we become allergic to a particular food
is by eating too much of it at one time. Our digestive
enzymes are not meant to handle mounds of mashed
potatoes or three glasses of milk at one sitting. When we
overeat a food, we use up the specific enzymes necessary for the digestion of that food. The food does not
digest as well, and an allergic reaction can result. Even
a healthful plate of vegetables can be troublesome to
digest if you eat more than you have the necessary
enzymes for. When you feel like indulging yourself, it
would be wise to go to the best buffet you can find and
eat tiny portions of many different foods.[5]

Improperly prepared foods can also cause allergic
reactions. Foods such as heated milk, chilled drinks,
overcooked foods, and fresh or cooked foods that have
been stored too long are difficult for the body to digest.
When protein is overcooked or overprocessed, the am-
monia level in the body increases, which can lead to a

toxic state in which nutrients cannot be easily used by the cells.[6]

All protein—whether meat, wheat, or vegetable protein—has the same chemical configuration. Over millions of years, we and our evolutionary ancestors developed enzymes that line up with protein molecules in our intestines. Protein has a heat labile point; at this temperature, the protein becomes denatured and undergoes a change in its chemical configuration. Because our enzymes are not designed to digest protein in an altered chemical state, we have trouble digesting such protein. Undigested noxious chemicals cross the intestinal membrane and get into the bloodstream, where the immune system is forced to deal with them. This may result in an allergic reaction.

Packaged and processed foods are also hard on the digestive system because they are made to sustain a long shelf life. The longer a food sits before it is eaten, the more depleted its nutrients become. Digestion is hindered by the absence of these nutrients. Unfortunately, processed foods replace the food value with substances the body cannot digest as well.

Some people find that their health, and their ability to digest food without allergic reaction, is never the same after a viral, bacterial, and/or parasitic infection. These infections, or the antibodies needed to combat the infections, seem to compromise the immune system. In many cases these people find themselves allergic to certain foods for the first time. Often these people become universal reactors, continually reacting to many items in their environment.

A healthy body is like an orchestra. Just as the different sections of an orchestra balance and enhance each other to create a harmonious sound, so to are the different parts of the endocrine system in a healthy body. The thyroid secretes thyroxin, the adrenals secrete adrenaline, and all of the glands secrete small amounts of hormones into the bloodstream so that a balance or harmony is maintained. When heredity, environmental factors, or illness upsets this balance, immune suppression occurs. The use of sugar, day in and day out, over a period of years—and eventually through several generations—can cause a certain degree of atrophy or abnormal functioning of the overworked glands. The more abnormal the functioning, the more upset the body chemistry, the more food sensitivities are likely to be present.

OTHER CAUSES OF ALLERGIES

Our polluted environment can also cause allergies. Studies show that city air may be three or four thousand times more polluted than sea air. Pollution from car exhaust, industrial waste, and pesticides can exacerbate food allergies. Indoor air pollution—at home and in the workplace—can add to the likelihood of environmentally triggered disease. One office was analyzed and found to have four hundred times greater concentrations of chemicals in the air as compared with the outside air. Each threshold limit was below the theoretically safe level for individual exposure to that particular chemical, but the combined and cumulative effects of multiple chemicals had never been evaluated.[7]

When a person is exposed to only one chemical, his or her body might be able to handle the toxin easily. However, when a person has to deal with chemicals from a variety of sources, this accumulation can become an overload, and may be too much for the body to handle effectively.

The environment of the average home has also been shown to be highly polluted. Fumes from gas heating and cooling appliances, the outgassing of such soft plastics as nylon, polyester, polyurethane, and polyethylene, and routine use of chemical-laden cleaning products all contribute to contamination. Another factor in the total overload of pollutants is the daily use of chemically contaminated water. A recent analysis of one city's local water system showed it to have 1,000 times more synthetic components than the average water system.[8]

A friend of mine who moved to England became allergic to almost everything in her environment within the first six months of living in her new home. Leaking pipes had caused gas to seep into the house. Once the gas company fixed the pipes, and the food allergens, which had accumulated over the previous six months, were removed from her diet, my friend slowly began to feel well again.[9]

Dr. William J. Rea found that some of his patients developed food allergies after they had been exposed to massive chemicals. Most of these patients could eat any food—as much and as often as desired—before they had been exposed to the chemicals. After exposure, it was apparent to many of the patients that foods, in general, bothered them. After unmasking the foods to which they were allergic and eliminating them from their diet, patients found that they were able to have symptom-free meals for the first time in months. In order to remain symptom free, it was clear that these patients had to continue avoiding their allergy-producing foods for a period of at least six to twelve months. As their exposure to chemicals decreased, their tolerance to foods increased, and they were able to eat foods previously not tolerated. Furthermore, during visits to areas of significantly lower air pollution, they found that they could tolerate foods to which they were usually susceptible. As you can see, there are no simple reasons why some people get food allergies, nor are there simple cures.[10]

Exposure to pollen, gases, hydrocarbons, animals, perfumes, and other substances can upset a person's body chemistry, but only when the body has already been compromised. A massive attack of any one substance can upset anyone's body chemistry; but, normal exposure to perfumes, paints, or newsprint generally will not upset a healthy person. When you remove sugar and the offending foods from your diet and stop further upsetting your chemistry through stress, your immune system will be rejuvenated and able to remove those offending allergens from your body easily.

WHAT'S AHEAD?

More research needs to be done to discover what happens to the body after the ingestion of different foods. Research designed to discover the impact of carbohydrate ingestion usually concerns itself with the rise and fall of blood glucose. Very little examination has been done on what happens to minerals, because very few clinicians today realize that minerals work only in relation to each other.

Much of the money that goes for research on food and disease comes from the food or the pharmaceutical industry. The food industry is not interested in supporting research on the effects of sugar on the body because it relies on sugar in the manufacturing of processed foods. And the pharmaceutical industry doesn't participate in non-drug-oriented research. In fact, sugar research would be harmful to the drug industry, because if people stopped eating sugar they wouldn't need so many drugs. Even the limited amount of experimentation in this field has launched a worldwide crusade toward whole foods and the virtual elimination of drugs.

So how exactly does this mineral-enzyme-allergy connection work? When protein is properly digested, it is first broken down into polypeptides and then into amino acids, which are absorbed in the bloodstream. When protein does not break down completely—when the enzymes charged with the job are incapable of performing properly due to a mineral deficiency—it can be absorbed through the intestinal wall and into the bloodstream, reaching tissue in partially digested form. The body's immune system correctly interprets this undigested or "putrefied" protein as foreign matter and goes on the attack, causing an allergic reaction.

In Chapter 4, we'll take a closer look at the complete allergy process, from acute reaction to chronic reaction to degenerative disease. Included are all of the typical symptoms of allergy, as well as addiction and the breakdown of the immune system. We'll also see how sugar works directly on the phagocytes (white blood cells of the immune system), decreasing their ability to absorb bacteria and fight off disease.

4
Destruction
of the
Immune System

In the 1930s, a researcher named Dr. Hans Selye began examining the effects of stress on the body. He observed that when people eat something to which they are allergic, or smell a chemical to which they are reactive, there is an initial alarm reaction—an acute reaction. If the stimulus continues, a stage of adaption follows, lasting from minutes to years. During this stage the symptoms are chronic. Finally, adaption fails and a stage of exhaustion is reached. In this degenerative stage the body enters a disease state and eventually dies.

In his book *Stress Without Distress*, Selye called this progression from the acute, to the chronic, and eventually to the degenerative stage, the Biological Stress Syndrome. This concept, which is only now being understood and acknowledged by the medical community, has come to be known as the General Adaptation Syndrome. There are many kinds of stress that can affect the body: stress from sugar, stress from food not properly digested, stress from a body out of alignment, and psychological stress, among others.[1]

Cigarette smoking is a good example of an environmental stimulus that sends the body into the General Adaptation Syndrome. Many people get dizzy, perspire, and sometimes even throw up when they first start smoking. This is the alarm reaction; the body is signalling that it is allergic to the smoke. If the person continues to smoke in spite of this initial reaction, his or her body will eventually adapt and smoking will no longer cause these symptoms. In fact, it will begin to feel good to smoke. The smoker is becoming addicted.

The smoker's body becomes so accustomed to compensating for the allergy that it will go through withdrawal symptoms if the substance is taken away. Finally, often after years of abuse and overwork, the mechanisms responsible for adaption break down and become exhausted. The body is no longer able to protect itself from the harmful substance, and a disease condition develops. The particular condition depends on the genetic weaknesses of the individual; it could be a cancer condition, heart condition, lung condition, or a variety of other malfunctions or degenerative illnesses.

The same thing happens with food allergies. In the previous chapter we saw how a food allergy begins. The overuse of sugar and other foods to which we have become allergic causes a mineral malfunction, which, in turn, causes an enzyme malfunction. When enzymes are incapable of properly digesting food, bits of undigested protein are able to escape into the bloodstream. The immune system properly recognizes these proteins as intruders, and digests them just as it would digest a virus.

STAGES OF AN ALLERGIC REACTION

When the immune system becomes exhausted through overuse, the symptoms of allergic reaction appear. At this point, there can be an acute reaction such as hay fever, joint pain, headache, or fatigue. If the body continues to be exposed, it proceeds through the other stages of the degenerative disease process: chronic reactions and degenerative reactions. Let's take a closer look at each of these three stages and how they relate to Selye's theory of alarm, adaption, and exhaustion.

Stage I: Acute Reaction

As Dr. Selye pointed out, the body's first reaction to a foreign substance (and the body treats a food to which it is allergic as a foreign substance) is one of alarm, one of protection. This is an acute reaction, an immediate response to a foreign stimulus or substance. The immune system goes into action. The reaction is usually over quickly, and the body returns to homeostasis.[2]

When a food that cannot be properly digested is introduced into the body for the first time, the body cannot cope with it. In babies, this might be the cause of such problems as diarrhea, diaper rash, vomiting, and colic. A baby's first experience with homogenized milk, for example, might cause an alarm (protective) reaction resulting in the throwing up of the milk.

My daughter Laurie is the perfect example of this. I was able to breastfeed her for only a month. As my milk decreased, I needed to give her milk from a bottle. Every time she finished the bottle, the milk came right back up. The guilt that I felt because I could not feed her was painful, and I'm sure that she could sense my pain, which probably distressed her little body even further.

The doctor told me simply to give her another bottle after she had thrown up the contents of the first one. It didn't seem right to me even at the time, but I did it. The second bottle usually stayed down; her body was adapting to the milk to avoid starving. Throwing up was Laurie's acute reaction to the milk. And although she eventually adapted to the substance, other symptoms developed.

If a food to which the body is allergic is continually eaten, eventually the body will adapt to that food. The symptoms of acute reaction disappear, but this does not mean that all is well. The reactions have simply grown more complex and chronic.

Stage II: Chronic Reaction

As the body adapts to the foreign substance, the immune system continues to defend the body from undigested protein just as it would from bacteria or a virus. Since the white blood cells of the immune system are made of protein—protein which the body needs and is not getting in a usable form—the system cannot function correctly and soon becomes exhausted. The more the immune system is exposed to the undigested or partially digested food, the less able the white cells are to respond correctly to any "invader." The body becomes predisposed to developing disease conditions, both infectious and degenerative.

With the weakening of the white cells, the body's initial acute reaction to certain foods changes to a chronic one. Chronic signifies slow progress that continues for a long time. During a chronic reaction, it takes longer for the body to return to homeostasis than it does during an acute reaction (and sometimes the body doesn't return to homeostasis at all). Joint pains, migraine headaches that last for days, edema, and swollen legs and hands are all chronic reactions, and all can be caused by food allergies.[3]

Laurie, for example, had colic reactions every afternoon from the time she was six months to ten months old; her little body was protesting again, this time chronically. As an older child, she had all the symptoms of allergy: eczema, constant runny nose, and sneezing. Finally we eliminated milk and other foods to which she was allergic from her diet, and all the symptoms disappeared.

Unfortunately, chronic symptoms of food allergy are usually treated by the medical community with pain medication, tranquilizers, antidepressants, stimulants, anticonvulsants, diuretics, muscle relaxants, nutrients, and even surgical removal of symptom-producing tissue. The best cure, as I found with Laurie, is withdrawal from the offending foods. Nevertheless, each time a person eats these foods, he or she suppresses the immune system and eventually exhausts it.

Babies who are allergic to milk but are continually fed it over a period of time will eventually keep the milk down. Their resistance to the milk diminishes, and the original alarm reaction virtually disappears. This stage of adaption, which is relatively free of symptoms, can also become a stage of addiction. If these babies don't get milk on a daily basis, they can go through withdrawal symptoms.

In our society we tend to eat a few foods over and over again. Our diet is not varied. Our crops are not rotated. Because of refrigerators and freezers, we can eat the same foods all year. "Fast foods" all contain the same basic elements: wheat, eggs, milk, caffeine, corn, yeast, and, worst of all, sugar. After overeating these foods on a regular basis, a person can become allergy-addicted to some of them. Most of us don't even realize we're addicted; we just know that we feel better when we eat certain foods. Knowingly or unknowingly, those who are addicted time their meals and snacks in order to avoid the withdrawal symptoms that come from not eating those foods. Of course, as we have seen, each time we eat a food to which we've become allergic, we suppress our immune system and eventually exhaust it.

During the adaptive stage of food allergy, a person can have withdrawal symptoms from three hours to three days after exposure to the offensive substance if he or she is not exposed to it again. The body takes a long time to return to normal from its chronic reaction. The only way to avoid the discomfort of that withdrawal is to expose the body to that substance again, to drink that cup of coffee or can of soda pop, to keep the body in continual reaction. This applies not only to food allergies but to sugar, alcohol, cigarettes, caffeine, and other abusive substances.[4]

Many phobias, anxieties, and obsessions develop during the withdrawal phase of addiction. Brain allergies or inflammation in specific areas of the central nervous system can cause emotional reactions from minor to psychotic proportions. An addicted person can become angry, depressed, hyperactive, or withdrawn. When I was in this state, I used to get nervous, impatient, and was apt to fly off the handle at the slightest provocation. Sugar is as addictive as any drug. One common characteristic of sugar addiction is that one taste of the substance leads to a craving for more, the same way certain drugs create cravings. Some drugs upset the body's homeostasis mechanism so completely that, in a struggle to get back to normal, the addict can take only another dose of the same drug. The more you have, the more you want, and the more manufacturers will provide.[5]

During withdrawal from drugs or allergy-producing foods, acidosis can occur. Acidosis is that state of imbalance in which the body is more acid than alkaline. The body's enzyme functions are dependent not only on minerals but also on a narrow pH range (acid-alkaline balance). Therefore, acidosis reduces the enzyme function, which results in still more undigested protein and further allergic reaction. In this acid state, the undigested protein (also called peptides and endorphins) might actually initiate addiction because of druglike effects. Some people might recognize this as a feeling of mellowness, others as fatigue or sleepiness. Foods can definitely change how you function, how you think, and how you feel.

The more addicted a person becomes to the food, the more of that food he or she eats, and the more the body is forced to adapt. This leads to an exhaustion of the enzymes necessary for proper digestion, and of the immune system, causing the body to move from chronic reaction and adaption to degenerative reaction and a diseased condition.

Stage III: Degenerative Reaction

Degenerative disease indicates a worsening of physical or mental qualities. In the case of such degenerative diseases as cancer, arthritis, and heart disease, the cells and tissues change. The functions of some cells and tissues may be stopped altogether, and the body has a hard time returning to and maintaining homeostasis. Eventually the entire biochemical balance needed for health is destroyed, and continued imbalance is the cause of disease.

Our genetic blueprint decides which disease we will get according to our inherited weakness. My weakness is in my chest. Early in my life, I had pneumonia. In my teens, a large calcium deposit was removed from one of my lungs. After a few more bouts with pneumonia, I ended up with chronic bronchitis. I feel very fortunate that I was able to change my lifestyle. This change not only stopped the degenerative disease process in my lungs, it also turned the process around. I was able to eliminate all the phlegm from my chest, and my body healed itself.

The consequences of continual abuse during the degenerative stage are grave. Let's consider, for example, an individual who is allergic to milk. The body may have adapted to milk, but eventually this ability to adapt will become exhausted. This final exhaustion could be due to an overload in the body of stressors—possibly the person ate too many milk products at one time and overdosed, or drank milk during hay fever season and the two stressors were too much for the body to handle. Milk had been suppressing the body's immune system for a long time, and the individual may have been exposed to excessive heat or cold, fatigue, infection, or emotional stress.

Signs that initially appeared after drinking milk, or possibly different signs, will reappear. They might take the form of joint pains, bloating, gas, or headaches. If this person does not stop drinking milk or eating milk products, or continues other dietary indiscretions and lifestyle abuses, the symptoms will become irreversible. Depending on the affected organs, determined by a person's genetic blueprint, the result could be death. You may never have heard of anyone dying of a milk allergy, but in some cases, the allergy has so worn down the immune system that the body becomes susceptible to other diseases.

The degenerative disease process now begins due to any of a number of problems such as acidosis, lack of protein, insufficient enzymes, an exhausted immune system, or cytotoxic reactions.

The stages of the allergy process—alarm, adaption and addiction, and exhaustion—are the same for any lifestyle abuse. If you don't stop doing the things that make your body sick, all the medicine, vitamins, and other nutritional supplements in the world won't make you well.

OTHER STUDIES

Two different research projects that evaluate the effects of sugar on the phagocytic index have been done at Loma Linda University. The phagocytes are those white blood cells of the immune system that eat up foreign invaders and debris; they are the Pac-Men of the body. The more bacteria eaten by each phagocyte, the stronger the immune system becomes and the less chance the body has of becoming diseased. The phagocytic index indicates the average number of invaders engulfed by a phagocyte.

One of the Loma Linda studies, conducted in 1973, examined the effects of sugar (sucrose), glucose, fructose, honey, orange juice, and starch on the phagocytic index. Except for the starch, all the substances were simple sugars. The starch was the only substance to cause a rise in the phagocytic index—the phagocytes actually ate up more bacteria after starch was ingested. The index was highest approximately thirty minutes after the volunteers ate the starch. The sugars, on the other hand, caused the phagocytic index to decrease greatly. The index was lowest two hours after ingestion.[6] In other words, the sugar had a negative effect on the amount of bacteria removed by the immune system. The graph in Figure 4.1 shows the reaction of phagocytes to starch and sugar.

Next, the researchers investigated the effect of fasting on the phagocytic index. After the subjects fasted for sixty hours, the phagocytic capacity to engulf foreign invaders rose from 11 per phagocyte to 16. Fasting appeared to strengthen the immune system, as shown in Figure 4.2.[7] The researchers did not check for food allergens, but if they had, and had removed them from the diets of these volunteers, the phagocytic index might have been as high before fasting as it was after.

These results correspond to the findings of an earlier Loma Linda study conducted in 1964, which proved that the higher the fasting blood glucose in diabetics, the lower the phagocytic index. Diabetes is a chronic condition characterized by an inability of the body to metabolize sugar properly. Even when fasting, diabetics have higher blood glucose than nondiabetics, and this excess glucose in the blood works to suppress the immune system. As a result, statistics show that diabetics are more susceptible to developing certain disease conditions than nondiabetics; they are more likely to have heart and blood problems, kidney and liver dysfunction, and eye problems, as well as infectious diseases.

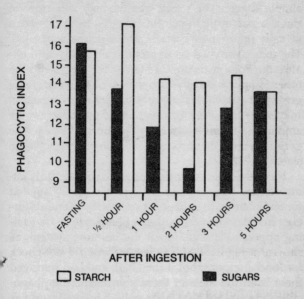

Figure 4.1. **Reaction of Phagocytes to Starch and Sugars**

These researchers also studied the actions of individual phagocytes under a microscope to observe the specific changes that occurred in the presence of sugar. Where the glucose level was normal, the phagocytic cells were very active. Pseudopods (little arms that reach out from the cell) extended in all directions in search of foreign objects. The higher the amount of sugar in the blood, however, the less active the cells became. An increased amount of fat was observed in the cells, resulting in slow, sluggish action of the phagocytes toward foreign objects.[8]

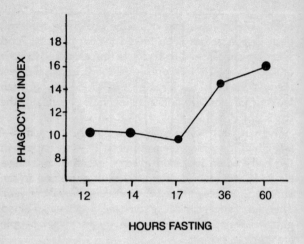

Figure 4.2.   **Effect of Fasting on Phagocytic Index**

RECENT INFORMATION

In 1912, Frenchman Louis Maillard discovered the reason
that some foods discolor and toughen when they are
cooked is due to a chemical attachment of the sugar (glucose) in the food to protein. This process, known as the
Maillard Reaction, causes toast to turn brown and steak to
toughen during cooking. High temperature causes this
binding of the glucose and protein molecules. Maillard
concluded that this reaction changes the structure of the
protein, making it difficult for the newly structured food
to be digested, assimilated, and metabolized by the body.
Besides barbecuing and frying foods, most processed
foods are heated to high temperatures, and the Maillard
Reaction is a problem for any food heated this way.

Recently, further research has been done on the Maillard Reaction (also known as the browning reaction) because cancer has been linked to this process. Food scientists are continually trying to find a method to slow or stop this reaction in processed food. To me, the best idea would be to avoid eating such foods rather than looking for a magic potion or formula to prevent the reaction.

New research has shown that this same reaction—sugar binding with protein abnormally—can happen in the body when its blood glucose becomes and stays elevated.[9] As stated earlier, the average person in the United States consumes 149 pounds of sugar per year. This glut of sugar can cause some to have elevated blood glucose levels, much more than in the past when people ate much less sugar.

When our blood and our blood cells are continually flowing with sugar, the sugar can bind nonenzymatically with protein. This may not sound very harmful, but it is. There is a normal process in which sugar binds enzymatically to protein in our body and forms glycoproteins, which are essential for our bodies to work properly. All of these chemical reactions in living tissues are under strict enzymatic control and conform to a tightly regulated metabolic program. When enzymes attach glucose to proteins, they do so at a specific site on a specific molecule for a specific purpose. Sugar and protein are not supposed to bind nonenzymatically, and if they do, glycated protein results. This process called glycation can permanently alter the molecular structure of the protein and, as a result, alter the way these glycated proteins or Advanced Glycated Proteins (AGEs) function in the body. The protein becomes toxic, resulting in cells that do not function optimally. This damages the body and exhausts the immune system. Eventually, degeneration occurs. Such changes can start as minor disturbances or disabilities and lead to specific illnesses.

This damage to the proteins takes place in two stages. The first product that is formed when glucose attacks protein is called a Schiff's base, which stays in the body for a few days. The Schiff's base is unstable and undergoes a slow chemical rearrangement that lasts several weeks until it forms a more stable union, the Amadori products. Amadori products undergo further chemical reactions until they form AGEs, which are irreversible. AGEs are characterized as brown or fluorescent pigments that seem to promote many age-related complications, such as atherosclerosis, hypertension, cataracts, and joint stiffness—common among diabetics, a group that chronically suffers from an excess of sugar in the blood.[10]

Glycation of blood proteins takes place when the levels of glucose shoot up and stay high. Anyone who drinks just one soft drink or eats a candy bar or donut on an empty stomach will find that their blood glucose levels shoot up.[11] The average person living in the United States today drinks over 450 sugary 12-ounce soft drinks per person per year.[12] Each soft drink contains approximately 10 teaspoons of sugar, so each person is getting over ¼ cup of sugar each day just from soft drinks. The average person consumes over ½ cup of sugar a day. This excess can bombard the blood with sugar much of the time, resulting in negative ramifications such as a suppressed immune system. This is certainly another reason to remove as much sugar from your diet as possible, and as soon as possible.

These studies addressed themselves to the problems of sugar in the diet. In this book I focus specifically on

Sugar Shock

In 1976, the sugar industry discovered it was cheaper to make sugar from corn than from beets or cane. Since then, high fructose corn syrup (HFCS) has replaced sucrose as a sweetener in most soft drinks, baked goods, and processed foods. Among other consequences, fructose has been implicated in heart disease, elevated blood cholesterol levels, and blood clotting. Worst of all, fructose causes the white blood cells of the immune system to become "sleepy" and unable to defend against harmful foreign invaders.

So stay away from that packaged white crystal-like stuff that you see in health food and grocery stores, and any food that has fructose, dextrose, dextrine, corn syrup, or HFCS on its ingredient label. It's a killer!

the effect of sugar on mineral relationships. The Loma Linda researchers looked at sugar's effect on the immune system. Maillard studied the binding of sugar with protein, while other researchers followed up with studies on glycation. Our conclusions are the same. Through the combined effects of mineral imbalance, allergic reaction, and phagocytic suppression, sugar can destroy the immune system and slowly but surely lead to degenerative disease.

In the next chapter we'll take a closer look at these degenerative diseases.

5
The
Consequences

The current life expectancy in the United States is over seventy-four years,[1] up from forty-nine years at the turn of the century.[2] This increase may seem miraculous, but those extra years have been almost wholly gained in the early years of life. Improved hospital conditions have reduced the number of deaths at birth, while advances in the medical field have brought infectious diseases such as polio, chicken pox, and measles under control. When these figures are included, the "average" person appears to live longer. However, when the extra years of early life are removed from the equation, the life expectancy of the average sixty-year-old male today is only two-and-a-half years longer than it was a hundred years ago. That is, once a male has attained the age of sixty, all the achievements of modern medicine extend his life only two-and-a-half years over his counterpart of a century ago. In terms of diseases of older people—arthritis, cancer, heart disease, diabetes, and others—not much headway has been made.

In the previous chapters we have seen how sugar goes about unbalancing the body's mineral relationships and weakening its immune system. This damage from sugar manifests itself in many degenerative diseases and harmful conditions. Those discussed briefly in this chapter are: hypoglycemia, hyperglycemia (diabetes), constipation, intestinal gas, asthma, headaches, psoriasis, cancer, arthritis, premenstrual syndrome, candidiasis, obesity, heart disease, osteoporosis, tooth decay, multiple sclerosis, inflammatory bowel disease, canker sores, gallstones, kidney stones, and cystic fibrosis.

It should be noted that these conditions in their less-serious stages can degrade the quality of one's life, producing feelings of, "I don't really feel well, but I'm not really sick." To whatever extent these conditions affect you, that extent can be greatly decreased by a healthy diet and lifestyle.

HYPOGLYCEMIA

The first organ of the endocrine system to come into contact with ingested foods or chemicals is the pancreas. Insulin, a hormone secreted by the pancreas, is responsible for controlling the amount of sugar in the bloodstream. Malfunctioning of the pancreas can cause either excessively low or abnormally high levels of sugar in the blood. Therefore, it is not surprising that of all the endocrine glands, the pancreas is the most susceptible to damage by excess sugar.

When we ingest sugar, our blood sugar level goes up. Clusters of endocrine cells in the pancreas, called the islets of Langerhans, detect this excess sugar in the blood and secrete insulin, which brings the blood sugar level back to normal. When sugar is eaten and overeaten obsessively for a number of years, the pancreas can become overstimulated and secrete too much insulin. Excess insulin can make the blood sugar drop below normal, and hypoglycemia (low blood sugar) may develop. Chromium is needed to digest sugar and many people deplete their store of chromium, which upsets all the mineral relationships.[3]

Pure sucrose and fructose are both metabolized to glucose and are rapidly absorbed. Because the hypothalamus is highly sensitive to changes in blood sugar, there is an endocrine reflex, causing the release of insulin. The brain adapts to a constant intake of sugar and becomes increasingly sensitive to virtually all kinds of stimuli. It is probably this hyper-reflex that is responsible for the hypoglycemic reactions common in sugar addicts.[4]

In addition to insulin, the islets of Langerhans secrete another hormone called glucagon, which stimulates the release of glycogen, a sugar stored in the liver and tissues. If this mechanism wears out from overuse, glycogen may not be released; this causes the individual to go into a hypoglycemic state. To compensate, the person may crave and eat more sugar to keep the blood sugar level normal, which, in turn, causes further destruction.

An interesting phenomenon that many physicians have discovered is that abnormally high (hyperglycemia) or abnormally low (hypoglycemia) blood sugar levels can occur in a person who has eaten a food or has come in contact with a chemical to which he or she is sensitive. These can include fats, carbohydrates, proteins, inhalants, and tobacco, and are specific to each individual. When the allergy-provoking substance is removed, the blood sugar level returns to normal.[5]

Hypoglycemia is considered the adaptive stage of

this allergic reaction; as the endocrine cells adapt to excess sugar or allergic substances, they begin to secrete too much insulin. Symptoms that might occur during a hypoglycemic state include fatigue (usually a few hours after sugar is ingested), falling asleep after meals, memory failure, rapid heartbeat, anxiety, tremors, hunger pangs, giddiness, headache, perspiration, and depression.

Although it was a long time ago, I can vividly remember driving home one day after having lunch with a friend. I began feeling weak and dizzy, and I was perspiring heavily. After lunch, along with a few cups of coffee, I had eaten a meringue dessert. I didn't think I had eaten enough sugar to produce such a strong reaction. What I hadn't realized, though, is when the homeostatic mechanisms of the body aren't working correctly, the caffeine in coffee, as well as sugar, can cause the blood sugar level to drop. So between the coffee and the meringue, I was in bad shape. These symptoms of hypoglycemia are not very pleasant, yet many people experience them day after day without really dealing with their cause. Many convince themselves that the symptoms are in their heads, while others feel they must learn to live with them. In fact, simply eliminating the junk food from your diet is a great start toward removing these symptoms. As scary as these symptoms are, what's even more scary is what this abusive dietary lifestyle does internally to the immune system, the glands, and the organs of the body.

DIABETES

If hypoglycemia is the adaptive stage of an allergic reaction, then hyperglycemia (diabetes) is the exhaustive stage. As with other overstimulated tissues and organs, the overworked pancreas eventually wears out and stops functioning correctly. The islets of Langerhans become exhausted and slow down or stop the secretion of insulin. The body can no longer adapt, as seen in hypoglycemia, and diabetes is the result.

Even if the islets continue to secrete insulin at a normal rate, that insulin may be too weak to do any good. As explained in Chapter 2, sugar causes a calcium-phosphorus imbalance that renders the body less capable of breaking down proteins into amino acids—the essential building blocks of hormones. With less protein, insulin begins to diminish; the resulting insulin deficiency can also cause hyperglycemia and diabetes.

There are two types of diabetes. The first, juvenile onset or Type-1 diabetes, is characterized by a complete lack of insulin in the islets of Langerhans. "Juvenile onset" doesn't mean that only children can get it; adults, too, can get this type of diabetes. There is a possibility that Type-1 is transmitted by a virus. Ten percent of all diabetics have Type-1 diabetes.[6]

Far more common is adult-onset or Type-2 diabetes, which is the type we will be concentrating on here. In Type-2 diabetics, although insulin is in the cells of the islets of Langerhans, an insufficient amount is secreted. And the insulin being secreted is either of poor quality, or it is unable to be used properly by the body. The mechanism for moving the insulin out of the cells and into the bloodstream has malfunctioned, and the levels of glucose in the blood remain high after a carbohydrate has been ingested. Some Type-2 diabetics have symptoms similar to Type-1—frequent urination, extreme thirst, ravenous hunger, weight loss, extreme fatigue, loss of concentration, memory failure, dizziness, unprovoked anxiety, tremors, cuts that are slow to heal, frequent skin infections, headaches—while others display no symptoms at all.[7]

Research shows that as sugar in the diet increases, there is an increased urinary excretion of chromium. Many diabetics have shown to be deficient in chromium. When this happens, other minerals cannot function as well.[8]

Many doctors today don't feel there is a correlation between how much sugar one eats and diabetes; but, as sugar consumption has increased in the United States, so has diabetes proportionally. During World War II, when sugar consumption dropped, the outbreak of diabetes dropped sharply also.

Dr. William Philpott helped many diabetics by finding the foods to which they had reactions and eliminating those foods from their diets. Many Type-2 diabetics needed little or no insulin once they had removed the reactive foods from their diets.[9]

In another experiment, a group of volunteers increased their sugar consumption to 40 percent of their diets for six weeks. Testing of their blood sugar levels and insulin levels before and after the six weeks showed higher levels of glucose and insulin, both while fasting and after sugar ingestion. Clearly, then, the mechanism that controls blood glucose becomes faulty when there are high levels of sugar in the diet.

The overeating of concentrated refined foods, including sugar and white flour, puts added strain on the pancreas and the production of insulin. Sugar goes into the bloodstream quickly. The more refined foods that are ingested, the greater the danger to the pancreas. It may take as long as twenty years for diabetes to develop. Maintaining normal weight, exercising, staying away from foods to which one is reactive, and eliminating refined sugar from the diet are four simple steps in helping to control Type-2 diabetes.[10]

CONSTIPATION

Not only does sugar put a strain on the pancreas, it has ramifications for other endocrine glands as well. When we continually overeat sugar and our blood sugar rises, the insulin level in our blood also rises. The thyroid gland must secrete the hormone thyroxin into the bloodstream to open the receptor cells and allow insulin into the cells. Eventually the thyroid itself becomes exhausted, and since the thyroid regulates metabolic functions, everything in the body slows down. Nutrient-rich blood moves through the body slowly. Blood pressure is lowered, making it more difficult for nutrients to move through the body. Feces also moves through the body slowly, commonly causing constipation.

Eating sugar over and over can lead to constipation in other ways. We've seen how sugar inhibits enzymes, and when enzymes aren't working properly, undigested food putrifies in the small intestine. Inflammation sets in to protect the lining of the small intestine and colon from the undigested proteins. This inflammation makes the passage smaller and more difficult for the feces to move through, and the mucus that forms makes it nearly impossible for nutrients to reach the bloodstream.

If sugar and white flour are a large part of your diet, you're lacking proper nutrients as well as fiber and bulk. Lack of fiber has been implicated in colon cancer because it allows feces to stay in the colon too long, and the bacteria that are supposed to be quickly eliminated from the body are not. The bacteria seep back into the walls of the colon and become toxic to the body. When there is no fiber to create bulk, the feces become hard and do not move along quickly through the colon. Hard feces can stick to the lining of the colon and cause diverticulitis, colitis, hiatal hernias, hemorrhoids, varicose veins, and other diseases.[11]

If you are suffering from constipation, you might consider making the following changes in your diet:

❑ Eliminate all refined foods.

❑ Eat lots of raw vegetables.

❑ Exercise (preferably aerobics) at least twenty minutes a day, five days a week.

❑ Drink six to eight 8-ounce glasses of water daily.

❑ Do not neglect the "calls of nature." You might find that half an hour later, nature is no longer calling.

❑ Eat only a small amount of animal protein at any one meal and chew it thoroughly. This will provide less opportunity for protein to putrify in the colon.

❑ Iron supplements such as iron sulfate and iron gluconate can cause constipation. If you need iron and are experiencing constipation, try a different form of iron supplementation such as ferrous fumerate or carbonyl iron.

❑ Avoid all commercial laxatives. Use herbal laxatives that include senna pods or senna leaves, flax, psyllium seed, or cascara sagrada. Herbal laxatives are sold in health food stores.

❑ Avoid coffee, tea, and alcohol. They have been found to cause constipation in many people.

❑ Take two tablespoons of vegetable oil a day (preferably cold-pressed) either plain or on a salad.

❑ Eat a high-fiber diet. There are three types of fiber: bran, pectin, and guar. Make sure your diet includes bran from whole grains, pectin from fruits, and guar from beans. Also, be sure to eat root and leafy green vegetables.

❑ Remove any foods to which you are allergic from your diet; they do not digest well.

There are many colon cleansing programs on the market. Some programs consist of bulking agents, herbs, vitamins, and minerals—all of which help to pull putrefied materials from the colon. Other programs include topical creams to stimulate the colon. Still other programs suggest taking enzymes at meals to prevent putrefied foods from collecting in the colon.

Many of these cleansing programs are effective. Keep two things in mind when deciding which program to use. The first is that most programs recommend fruit juice. You can simply substitute the fruit juice with vegetable juice or spring water. The second thing to remember is that you might be allergic to one of the items in the program. Test each supplement individually and check your body's reaction. Take one in the morning on an empty stomach. Take your pulse before taking the supplement and ten minutes after you have taken it to see if your pulse rate increases or decreases ten beats per minute; if so, this is an indication of a sensitivity. Watch for symptoms during the first hour. If you have a Body Chemistry Test Kit (see page 161), take the calcium-urine test to discover any sensitivities.

Don't forget that if you resume the consumption of refined foods, your colon can become clogged again. Concentrate on changing your dietary habits to keep your body in harmony and functioning optimally.

How Sugar and Sweeteners Can Ruin Your Health

Lick the Sugar Habit warns of the negative—often dangerous—effects of sugar on the body. In addition to throwing off the body's homeostasis, excess sugar may result in a number of other significant consequences. Using documentation from a variety of medical journals and other scientific publications, I have summed up the consequences of a body out of homeostasis due to eating excess sugar. You might make a copy of this list and put it on your refrigerator or tape it to the pantry door where you keep your sugar bowl.

- *Sugar can suppress the immune system.*[1]
- *Sugar can upset the body's mineral balance.*[2]
- *Sugar can cause hyperactivity, anxiety, concentration difficulties, and crankiness in children.*[3]
- *Sugar can cause drowsiness and decreased activity in children.*[4]
- *Sugar can adversely affect children's school grades.*[5]
- *Sugar can produce a significant rise in triglycerides.*[6]
- *Sugar contributes to a weakened defense against bacterial infection.*[7]
- *Sugar can cause kidney damage.*[8]

■ *Sugar can reduce helpful high density lipoproteins (HDLs).*[9]

■ *Sugar can promote an elevation of harmful low density lipoproteins (LDLs).*[10]

■ *Sugar may lead to chromium deficiency.*[11]

■ *Sugar can cause copper deficiency.*[12]

■ *Sugar interferes with absorption of calcium and magnesium.*[13]

■ *Sugar may lead to cancer of the breast, ovaries, prostate, and rectum.*[14]

■ *Sugar can cause colon cancer, with an increased risk in women.*[15]

■ *Sugar can be a risk factor in gall bladder cancer.*[16]

■ *Sugar can increase fasting levels of glucose.*[17]

■ *Sugar can weaken eyesight.*[18]

■ *Sugar raises the level of a neurotransmitter called serotonin, which can narrow blood vessels.*[19]

■ *Sugar can cause hypoglycemia.*[20]

■ *Sugar can produce an acidic stomach.*[21]

■ *Sugar can raise adrenaline levels in children.*[22]

■ *Sugar malabsorption is common in those with functional bowel disease.*[23]

■ *Sugar can speed the aging process, causing wrinkles and grey hair.*[24]

■ *Sugar can lead to alcoholism.*[25]

■ *Sugar can promote tooth decay.*[26]

■ *Sugar can contribute to weight gain and obesity.*[27]

- *High intake of sugar increases the risk of Crohn's disease and ulcerative colitis.*[28]

- *Sugar can cause a raw, inflamed intestinal tract in persons with gastric or duodenal ulcers.*[29]

- *Sugar can cause arthritis.*[30]

- *Sugar can cause asthma.*[31]

- *Sugar can cause candidiasis (yeast infection).*[32]

- *Sugar can lead to the formation of gallstones.*[33]

- *Sugar can lead to the formation of kidney stones.*[34]

- *Sugar can cause ischemic heart disease.*[35]

- *Sugar can cause appendicitis.*[36]

- *Sugar can exacerbate the symptoms of multiple sclerosis.*[37]

- *Sugar can indirectly cause hemorrhoids.*[38]

- *Sugar can cause varicose veins.*[39]

- *Sugar can elevate glucose and insulin responses in oral contraception users.*[40]

- *Sugar can lead to periodontal disease.*[41]

- *Sugar can contribute to osteoporosis.*[42]

- *Sugar contributes to saliva acidity.*[43]

- *Sugar can cause a decrease in insulin sensitivity.*[44]

- *Sugar leads to decreased glucose tolerance.*[45]

- *Sugar can decrease growth hormone.*[46]

- *Sugar can increase cholesterol.*[47]

- *Sugar can increase systolic blood pressure.*[48]

- *Sugar can change the structure of protein, causing interference with protein absorption.*[49]

- *Sugar causes food allergies.*[50]
- *Sugar can contribute to diabetes.*[51]
- *Sugar can cause toxemia during pregnancy.*[52]
- *Sugar can contribute to eczema in children.*[53]
- *Sugar can cause cardiovascular disease.*[54]
- *Sugar can impair the structure of DNA.*[55]
- *Sugar can cause cataracts.*[56]
- *Sugar can cause emphysema.*[57]
- *Sugar can cause atherosclerosis.*[58]
- *Sugar can cause free radical formation in the bloodstream.*[59]
- *Sugar lowers the enzymes' ability to function.*[60]
- *Sugar can cause loss of tissue elasticity and function.*[61]
- *Sugar can cause liver cells to divide, increasing the size of the liver.*[62]
- *Sugar can increase the amount of fat in the liver.*[63]
- *Sugar can increase kidney size and produce pathological changes in the kidney.*[64]
- *Sugar can overstress the pancreas, causing damage.*[65]
- *Sugar can increase the body's fluid retention.*[66]
- *Sugar can cause constipation.*[67]
- *Sugar can cause myopia (nearsightedness).*[68]
- *Sugar can compromise the lining of the capillaries.*[69]
- *Sugar can cause tendons to become brittle.*[70]
- *Sugar can cause headaches, including migraines.*[71]

- ■ *Sugar can cause an increase in delta, alpha, and theta brain waves, which can alter the mind's ability to think clearly.* [72]

- ■ *Sugar can cause depression.* [73]

- ■ *Sugar can increase insulin responses in those consuming high-sugar diets compared to low-sugar diets.* [74]

- ■ *Sugar increases bacterial fermentation in the colon.* [75]

- ■ *Sugar can cause hormonal imbalance.* [76]

- ■ *Sugar can cause blood platelet adhesiveness, which causes blood clots.*

STOMACH OR INTESTINAL GAS

Gas forms whenever food does not digest properly; it is, therefore, another clear signal of an unbalanced body chemistry. Stomach gas is usually caused by too much or too little hydrochloric acid in the stomach. If gas occurs immediately after swallowing the food, this indicates that the stomach has a high level of hydrochloric acid. If gas forms from one to several hours later, or it is present the morning after eating the food, a deficiency in hydrochloric acid is indicated. Intestinal gas can also be due to disturbed liver and pancreatic functions. An overactive liver or an underactive pancreas makes for an acidic stool; whenever stools are too alkaline or too acidic, gas is produced.

If gas is a problem for you, the following suggestions may help to correct it:

❑ Limit your protein intake to no more than two ounces for any meal.

❑ Eat meals slowly.
❑ Eliminate foods—such as beans (especially baked and lima), onions, radishes, turnips, yams, parsnips, lettuce hearts, and sugar—which are known to cause gas in some people.
❑ Chew each bite of food well, at least twenty times.
❑ Eat fruit between meals only.

Many foods to which you are allergic can cause gas. You can check for these reactive foods by taking the calcium-urine test found in the Body Chemistry Test Kit (see page 161). Once you have identified these foods, eliminate them from your diet.

ARTHRITIS

Arthritis is a painful inflammatory disease of the joints and bones. Rheumatoid arthritis and osteoarthritis are the two major types. Rheumatoid arthritis is an inflammation of the body's synovial joints. Osteoarthritis involves deterioration of the cartilage that covers the ends of the bones.[12]

There is considerable evidence that people who are allergic to certain foods build immune complexes in their blood. These immune complexes are a combination of food to which we are allergic and a protective substance called an antibody, which our body makes to defend us against what the body considers a foreign invader. As these foreign substances are glued together by the antibodies, an immune complex develops. These complexes, which often collect in the joints, cause tissue damage and inflammation, partly from the release of free radicals, the by-product of the immune complexes.

A food allergy does not develop unless a body is out of homeostasis. A body that has been compromised due to mineral imbalance is unable to make enzymes to remove the free radicals from the body. Inflammation in the bones, joints, and cartilage can be caused by an accumulation of toxic minerals, mostly calcium. This, too, is caused by a body out of balance.[13]

Dr. William Catterall points out in an article in *Arthritis News Today* that in over 232 cases from four independent investigators, in which the diets of arthritis patients were carefully controlled, the following observations were made:

• With few exceptions, when a restricted (or fasting) diet was followed, acute arthritic symptoms disappeared.

• Arthritic symptoms returned when certain foods were individually reintroduced to the diet.

• The symptoms disappeared again when each one of such foods was withdrawn.

• Most patients experienced several cycles of symptom production and remission in response to certain foods.

The connection between arthritic symptoms and ingestion of offending foods was forcefully and repeatedly demonstrated.[14 15]

Arthritic patients often experience symptoms such as fatigue, weakness, and fever, which are also symptomatic of allergy addiction and withdrawal. Food allergy symptoms in many people get worse during the night or early in the morning, perhaps accounting for arthritic morning stiffness.

Once again we see that if we eliminate the substances that upset the body, the body will heal itself.

ASTHMA

An asthma attack is caused by spasms in the muscles that surround the bronchi (small airways in the lungs), constricting the outward passage of air. Typical symptoms of an asthma attack include coughing, wheezing, a feeling of tightness in the chest, and difficulty in breathing.[16]

Asthmatic attacks have been ascribed to three main causes: allergy, infection, and emotional disturbance. Recent research has shown that food allergy plays a large role.

A study conducted in Israel indicated that of twenty-two patients with asthma, fifteen improved remarkably within weeks after avoiding all dairy foods. When the fifteen patients were then challenged with dairy products, five had a recurrence of severe asthma attacks.[17] Unfortunately, the study didn't test the patients for other food allergies, which are individual to each person. With further investigation, more of the study subjects may have been helped.

Researchers involved in a year-long study concluded that the involvement of allergic foods in those with bronchial asthma is more frequent than previously believed. Of the ninety-five subjects, 98 percent showed a distinct decrease of asthmatic complaints with the avoidance of allergic foods for six to twelve months.[18]

Detective work for asthmatics involves extensive research because three types of bronchial responses must be observed: immediate responses (onset within twenty to forty-five minutes, with resolution within two hours after food challenge), late response (onset within four to six hours, resolving within twenty-four hours), and delayed type (onset within twenty-eight to thirty-two hours, resolving within forty-eight to fifty-six hours after food challenge). An asthmatic might best work with a clinician to help with this detective work.[19]

HEADACHES

Over the years, many studies have been done to establish a link between foods and headaches. For instance, caffeine has been implicated because it restricts the blood vessels. Tyramine-containing foods—including cheese, organ meats, alcohol, chocolate, yogurt, and smoked and aged meats—have also been suggested as headache causes.[20] Monosodium glutamate (MSG), a substance commonly used as a flavor enhancer in many processed foods and Oriental-style dishes has been implicated in a variety of symptoms including headaches.[21]

In a recent study done at Charing Cross Hospital in London, cooked wheat was found to cause headaches in 78 percent of the people tested, orange juice in 65 percent, cooked eggs in 45 percent, tea and coffee in 40 percent, chocolate and pasteurized milk in 37 percent, beef in 35 percent, and corn, cane sugar, and yeast in 3 percent each. When these common foods were avoided, there was a dramatic drop in the number of headaches experienced per month by the study subjects; 85 percent became headache-free.[22]

Research shows that many children with frequent headaches have an increased gut permeability. This means increased noxious substances, which include undigested or partially digested food, are more readily absorbed in the permeable gut. This is believed to trigger headaches.[23]

Through my professional experience, I believe that

any food can cause a headache. Moreover, symptoms do not follow the same pattern in each person; headaches may occur immediately after the reactive food has been eaten or up to twenty-four hours later. To discover the food or foods that may be causing the headaches, each must be tested individually. First, the food(s) must be withdrawn from the body for four days (a person may experience withdrawal symptoms for this period of time). At this point, the "suspect" foods should be reintroduced one at a time, and symptoms should be investigated through a blood test or a urine test (see the Body Chemistry Test Kit on page 161).

Remember, there are other common causes for headaches. Stress is one major contributor. Stress upsets the body chemistry, which can result in the improper digestion of food. In turn, the partially digested food enters the bloodstream, resulting in headaches in some people.

PSORIASIS

Psoriasis is a skin disease that manifests itself as large scaly patches that appear all over the body or in a specific area. Psoriasis is often an indication that the liver is not functioning correctly; therefore, a liver-cleansing program is a good place to start. The cleansing programs suggested for constipation (see page 67) can also be used for the liver. When the body chemistry has been compromised, it is important to to find out what is upsetting it.

Dr. John M. Douglass, with Kaiser Permanente Medical Group in Los Angeles, uses elimination diets to improve the conditions of his psoriasis patients. Douglass has his patients eliminate acidic foods and beverages, such as tomatoes, pineapple, coffee, and soda, from their diets. This results in great improvement.[24]

When the liver is functioning well and reactive foods have been eliminated from the diet, excellent results can be achieved. This is not, however, a rapid process. Although preliminary results can be seen within a few weeks, the program needs to be followed for many months.

CANCER

Statistics show that lifestyle is strongly associated with the incidence of cancer. Cancer is a condition in which normal cells turn abnormal and begin reproducing uncontrollably. It is clearly important to have some understanding of the process that causes cancer to occur. The theory that relies upon the nutritional ideas described in this book is given below. These ideas can greatly help you and your doctor battle cancer.

In the 1920s, early cancer research was done by Dr. Otto Walberg. In his investigation of human cells, he discovered that removing 35 percent of the oxygen from their environment caused the cells to become cancerous. When he put oxygen back into the cells, they did not return to normal. Further research has verified Dr. Walberg's beliefs.

One way in which cells turn cancerous is through a continually upset body chemistry. When the body chemistry is normal, cells develop poisonous by-products called free radicals. These include peroxide, hydroxyl group, and superoxide. A healthy body also produces enzymes—peroxidase, catalase, and superoxide dismutase—that treat these free radicals and turn them into useful products. Enzymes depend on minerals to function properly. For example, peroxidase is a selenium-dependent enzyme.[25]

If you continually cause body chemistry imbalance by eating sugar or other abusive foods, or if you stress your body by burning the candle at both ends or by constantly experiencing distress, anger, or rage, you will increase your metabolic rate and produce more free radicals. You will also inhibit peroxidase, superoxide dismutase, and catalase, allowing the free radicals to build up in your system.[26] A buildup of free radicals interferes with the oxygenation process, which, as seen earlier, can cause normal cells to turn cancerous.

The body strives to maintain homeostasis at all times. This can be seen in a homeostatic phenomenon that occurs in the cells called *contact inhibition*. When your body is injured—for example, if you have a cut—the healthy cells surrounding that cut reproduce to replace the ones that have been harmed. Through contact inhibition these cells know to stop producing once they have filled in the injured area. In other words, division stops when the cells become so numerous that they touch each other. It is believed that a chemical "messenger" that inhibits further cell division is passed from cell to cell. In contrast, cancer cells continue dividing even after cells touch. Thus, cancer cells appear to have lost the homeostatic mechanism of contact inhibition.[27]

Another factor involved in the cancer process is a person's genetic blueprint. If you were born with a genetic blueprint that caused your endocrine system to oversecrete estrogen, and you keep yourself healthy, you will be a healthy emotionally sensitive person. In addition, if you oversecrete growth hormone from a genetically overactive anterior pituitary, and you are healthy, you probably will likely be a big, sensitive person. If, however, through an abusive lifestyle, you continuously upset your body chemistry, you could start interfering with the oxygenation of your cells. Too much estrogen and growth hormone naturally found in the body, coupled with a lack of oxygen, could cause cells to become cancerous.

The most important thing to remember is this: When you upset your body chemistry often enough, many of your 63 trillion cells will not be able to oxygenate; they won't metabolize properly and will become toxic. The cells say, "Why should I function properly when you treat me like this?"

Cells that lifestyle abuses cause to turn cancerous develop a protective coating because they know they are going to be attacked by the immune system. The immune system is also being compromised by the person's lifestyle, which is why the body's cells turned cancerous in the first place. If a person does not change the abusive lifestyle that wears down his or her body, the sick cells will start winning—in other words, the cancer cells will be able to take over the body.

A person's genes do not cause disease—rather, the culprit is an abusive lifestyle that constantly upsets the body chemistry. We are all born with a genetic blueprint. When you upset your body chemistry continually, the disease of your genetic blueprint is more likely to develop than if you keep your body in balance. This concept forces us to recognize that we are responsible for our disease. It puts the monkey on our back.

OSTEOPOROSIS

Osteoporosis is a progressive disease in which the bones gradually weaken, making the individual susceptible to bone fractures. This rarification of bone is due to loss of minerals and protein matrix. As we have seen, sugar causes the body's phosphorus and calcium levels to either increase or decrease. Since all minerals work in relation to each other, only that calcium which is in the proper ratio to phosphorus is available to function properly in the body. Unfortunately, many doctors persist in treating osteoporosis as a simple calcium deficiency and prescribe calcium supplements. This might be helpful for those who have enough phosphorus in the blood to balance the extra calcium. However, if there is more calcium than can work in relation with the phosphorus, the supplemental calcium will not help at all. Instead, this excess calcium will become toxic and can cause such problems as bone spurs, arthritis, hardening of the arteries, kidney stones, gallstones, cataracts, and tooth plaque.

Stomach acid is another crucial factor in calcium absorption and, ultimately, bone health. Calcium is absorbed in the upper part of the small intestine, and acid is essential for this process. That's why the frequent use of antacids wreaks havoc on bones.[28] Stomach acid production decreases as we grow older and may be one of the reasons why the efficiency of calcium absorption declines with age. Children absorb 75 percent of the calcium they take in; adults absorb only 30 to 50 percent.

One look at the average American diet should be enough to see that most calcium deficiency is not due to a lack of calcium in the diet. We are getting more calcium than ever before by eating more calcium-rich milk products—milk shakes, cheese-topped pizzas and burgers, fruit yogurts, cheese-filled crêpes, ice cream, and cheesecake, to name a few. Although these products contain plenty of calcium, as well as other vitamins and minerals, the sugar that is also contained prevents the nutrients from being readily available.

When you eat ice cream, for example, you are certainly getting a healthy dose of calcium. However, the sugar in the ice cream alters the phosphorus in the blood, and much of the calcium can become toxic rather than useful. Even if the ice cream contained 400 milligrams of calcium, that calcium would metabolize incorrectly and either become toxic or be secreted in the urine. Milk products that include sugar can bring about a deficiency in the enzyme lactase, making the body unable to digest and absorb the milk. This can cause an allergic reaction to the milk. Each time you drink that milk or eat that food to which you are sensitive, you change your calcium-phosphorus ratio. Little calcium is assimilated from the milk or milk products, and the body must turn to its bones for the calcium and other minerals it needs. In other words, although a person drinks calcium-rich milk, if he or she is allergic to the milk and cannot utilize the calcium, the body will pull the calcium it needs from the bones, and that excess calcium can become toxic in the bloodstream.

Other substances in the diet can also affect the body's ability to absorb calcium. Caffeine, for example—just three cups of caffeinated coffee can make you excrete forty-five milligrams of calcium. The same thing happens with caffeinated tea and soft drinks. Even if the soft drink is sugar-free and caffeine-free, it still contains phosphoric acid, which also disrupts the calcium-phosphorus ratio.[29]

A correlation has also been found between cigarette smoking and osteoporosis. A number of recent studies have found that at least three-quarters of the women who develop osteoporosis are or were smokers (most smoke or smoked a pack or more a day).[30]

Certain medications, when used over a long period,

can also interfere with calcium availability. These medications include the blood thinner heparin, diuretics, aluminum-containing antacids, anticonvulsion medications, large doses of thyroid hormone, and corticosteroids.[31]

Excess sodium from salt causes excess calcium to be excreted in the urine. When calcium is excreted in urine, calcium blood levels drop. This causes the release of the parathyroid hormone, which breaks down bone in an effort to restore the level of calcium to the blood.[32]

A harmful substance that we don't think of in terms of food consumption is aluminum. Aluminum can enter the body through several sources: antacids, softened water, products such as cheese and pickles, cookware, food containers, foil (always remove the foil before eating a foil-covered baked potato—never poke your fork through the aluminum to get to the potato), and many deodorants and toothpastes. Aluminum, which is now being linked to Alzheimer's disease, can also decrease calcium absorption.[33]

Alcohol is yet another substance that can draw calcium from the bones. Used in excess, alcohol can seriously damage the body.[34]

Anything that inhibits the body's ability to absorb calcium contributes to the likelihood of osteoporosis. Sugar is the main dietary culprit—sugar eaten as a child, sugar eaten as a teenager, and sugar eaten in adulthood.[35] Osteoporosis starts slowly, usually with neckaches and/or back pain, and it may take decades for the disease to manifest itself. Chronic pain, the result of a phosphorus deficiency, soon sets in. A chiropractor may be needed over and over to keep the body aligned. Whenever calcium is taken from the bones, each time it is pulled across the cell membrane (such as when sugar is ingested), protein may be pulled as well. A lack of usable protein indicates that the tissues and bones are being compromised, and the disease progresses. At this stage, the slightest fall may cause a serious injury. A disc may rarefy, get spongy, and need to be removed. The simple task of reaching over to tie a shoe may cause a pinched nerve, resulting in inflammation; and since the body is unable to heal itself, that inflammation becomes a disease process. Doctors may be forced to use cortisone to stop the inflammation, and a vicious cycle begins.

All of these results, however, are reversible. Stop upsetting mineral relationships, and the body will heal itself. Personally, I have an easy way of knowing when my phosphorus is low and if I'm deficient in functioning calcium. When I wake up in the middle of the night or in the morning, I point my toes. If my legs or feet start to cramp, I know my body is low in calcium. This doesn't happen to everyone, but it certainly happens to me. And whenever it does, I think of the things I did and the foods I ate the day before, and try to figure out how I upset my mineral relationships.

Symptoms of calcium deficiency vary from person to person. Because calcium is necessary for many heart functions, some people experience palpitations when their functioning calcium level drops. Other common symptoms include insomnia, nervousness, arm and leg numbness, rheumatism, arthritis, menstrual cramps, premenstrual cramps, menopausal problems, nervousness, finger tremors, backaches, bone pain, soft nails, and tooth plaque.

Some forms of calcium are more easily digested than others. The most easily absorbed calcium supplements are calcium chelate, calcium orotate, and calcium ascorbate. Also, calcium is not readily taken in by the cell unless it is accompanied by magnesium. This is because the cell prefers to maintain a ratio of two parts of magnesium to every three parts of calcium. Thus, to offer to the cell membrane a straight calcium compound without magnesium is to ask it to alter its normal ratios, which it is not inclined to do. Therefore, the cell tends to reject the unescorted calcium, which is eliminated in the urine or stool. Today the preferred ratio of calcium to magnesium in a supplement is one to one. However, whether or not calcium supplementation prevents osteoporosis is debatable. Your best bet is to try to prevent it in the first place.[36]

Periodontal disease (pyorrhea) and gum disorders are forms of osteoporosis of the mouth. As a nutritional consultant, I see many people with osteoporosis of both the bones and of the mouth. In both cases, the patients secrete excess calcium in their urine. There is a simple test you can perform at home to see if you are doing the same (see Body Chemistry Test Kit on page 161). To combat periodontal disease, it is essential to stop using or consuming items that cause calcium to become deficient and/or toxic. This includes products such as ice cream, fruit yogurt, tea, coffee, cigarettes, and aluminum. A reduction in the amount of cooked protein eaten at one meal is also wise; people who have followed a vegetarian diet for twenty years or more, both men and women, show less bone loss than those who eat meat.[37] If you are allergic to milk products, it is wise to stop consuming them as well.

It is still possible to get plenty of calcium in your diet even if you must restrict your intake of milk and milk products. Other foods that are high in calcium include sardines, canned salmon, dark green leafy vegetables (spinach, collards, kale, turnip greens, mustard greens), broccoli, Brazil nuts, tofu and all soy products, sunflower seeds, and hulled sesame seeds. There is as much calcium in a glass of carrot juice as there is in a glass of milk; and the calcium in the carrot juice is more absorbable for many people. Remember—when your lifestyle keeps your minerals in good relationship and functioning efficiently, your body can easily absorb all of the nutrients in the food you eat. Many foods have small amounts of calcium, and a balanced body will be able to absorb all of it.

Exercise is the only way short of potent medication to significantly increase bone mass after you have stopped growing. As with muscles, stress (not distress) on the bones strengthens them. Activities that stress the long bones in the body, such as rope jumping, basketball, tennis, jogging, walking, rebounding on trampolines, cycling, and dancing are all effective in preventing osteoporosis. One study showed that postmenopausal women who exercised for one hour a day, three days a week for one year, actually gained body calcium, whereas a comparison group of sedentary women lost calcium.[38] And if you exercise outdoors in the sun, you will also be getting a good dose of vitamin D, which is needed for calcium absorption.

Recent findings indicate that estrogen may prevent osteoporosis in postmenopausal women;[39] however, this therapy is controversial. Women who are treated with small dosages of estrogen supplements continuously for ten to fifteen years are less likely to lose significant amounts of bone than women who do not take the supplements. Estrogen therapy does include some risks; it may promote the growth of a variety of cancers, including those of the uterine and breast in some women. To reduce the risk of cancer, estrogen is usually given in conjunction with progesterone, which helps mimic the natural premenopausal hormone cycle.

Still, many experts believe certain women should not take postmenopausal hormone therapy. Some women, for instance, through lifestyle excesses, have set the stage for increased risk of illness. Women who have fibrocystic breasts, those who have had cancer of the breast or the reproductive organs, and those who have a family history of these cancers are advised against taking hormonal therapy. My feeling is that Mother Nature did a good job of putting our bodies together. Why tinker with a good thing? Women who are considering hormonal therapy must give serious consideration to its risks along with the advantages.

The safest way, then, to stop bone loss and maintain adequate calcium in the body is to keep the minerals in balance through proper nutrition and exercise. Eliminate foods that upset the body chemistry, and avoid lifestyle excesses. I have seen postmenopausal women go from secreting calcium twenty-four hours a day to normal levels within a few weeks of following healthy lifestyle guidelines (see the program outlined in Chapter 9). It's the same story—lead a lifestyle that promotes a proper mineral balance and the body will heal itself.

HEART DISEASE

Heart and vascular disease resulting from lifestyle excesses and subconscious negative, stressful attitudes, affects one of every two persons in the United States. There is much research that indicates a link between a diet that includes sugar and heart disease.

The average daily sugar intake of patients with coronary and peripheral vascular diseases was found to be
higher—113 to 128 grams—than that of healthy subjects
in a control group, in which the average sugar intake
was 58 grams.[40] As researcher and author Dr. John Yudkin points out, "A person . . . who is taking more than
120 grams of sugar a day [4 ounces or 8 tablespoons or
24 teaspoons; a 12-ounce soft drink has 3 tablespoons]
(one of the major lifestyle excesses) is perhaps five or
more times as likely to develop myocardial infarction
[clotting of the coronary artery in the heart] as one taking
less than 60 grams."[41]

Much of this damage is due to sugar's unbalancing
of the body's chemistry and its mineral relationships.
Clinician and researcher Dr. William Philpott found
that people who die of coronary artery disease—arte-
riosclerosis—have no detectable amount of chromium in their aortas, while those who die accidentally
and manifest no coronary artery disease do have chromium in their aortas. This is directly attributable to
sugar; our bodies need chromium to digest sugar.
Since sugar contains no chromium, it must be leached
from the body.[42]

In a study that included eleven men, 10 percent
of the calories that they ate as fat were replaced by
glucose. There was a statistically significant increase of blood triglycerides and a decrease in high-
density lipoproteins.[43] High-density lipoproteins
protect us from heart disease.

Research presented on April 29, 1985, at the American Chemical Society's 189th national meeting in Miami, Florida, suggests that it is the quality of cholesterol
in the diet, not the quantity, that contributes most to the
risk of developing coronary heart disease and athero-

sclerosis (hardening of the arteries). In the past, conventional thought implicated a diet rich in fat with human heart disease. The research suggests that those natural fats might present a serious hazard only if and when they are transformed through oxidation (mainly from overcooking).[44]

Fred A. Kummerow, a food chemist for the University of Illinois, states that all lipids (fats) are unstable and will eventually oxidize. He also believes that cooking speeds the oxidation process. Kummerow showed that oxidized lipids are toxic to arterial cells.

In one in vitro cell test, both partially oxidized cholesterol and partially oxidized vitamin D (also a lipid) decreased the cells' ability to keep out nonfunctioning calcium. The researchers claim that in addition to killing cells, too much nonfunctioning calcium also creates deposits that characterize advanced atherosclerotic lesions.[45] Dr. Hans Selye found that he could stress rats and cause them heart disease, and then, by giving them extra magnesium and potassium, reduce some of the problem.[46] In my practice I have seen the normalization of blood pressure, cholesterol level, and triglyceride level of many people by removing the sugar and the foods to which they are sensitive from their diets. Your lifestyle and dietary excesses do have a direct impact on causing heart disease and, indeed, other degenerative diseases.

I have talked a lot about the calcium-phosphorus ratio and how it is upset by sugar intake. Current medical research has implicated both an excess and a deficiency of functioning calcium in heart disease. This certainly suggests, even to the untrained observer, that in order for calcium to be properly utilized, it must be in the right relationship with all other minerals.[47]

Through his studies on coronary artery disease, Dr. Philpott (page 88) also believes that magnesium, calcium, and chromium form a biochemical team that must be present in order for humans to resist degenerative disease.[48] Copper is another factor. Researchers McKenzie and Kay have demonstrated that individuals with hypertension excrete over two and a half times more copper in their urine than control groups with no hypertension.[49] Many see this as a correlation between a deficiency in functioning minerals and disease, but few connect this deficiency to undigested food and enzymes. In order to work properly, each one of the body's little enzymes needs different functioning minerals. When just one mineral is functionally deficient or toxic, the result is an upset body chemistry and an imbalance in all mineral relationships.

Many of you may have changed from sugar to fructose because of studies showing that fructose is absorbed only 40 percent as quickly as glucose and causes only a modest rise in blood sugar. Dr. J. Hallfrisch studied cholesterol and triglyceride levels and found that fructose, unfortunately, caused a general increase in both the total serum cholesterol level and the low-density lipoprotein fraction of cholesterol in most subjects. The triglyceride levels also rose significantly, especially in those persons whose blood sugar levels rise higher than normal when they eat sugar. It was concluded that high levels of dietary fructose can produce undesirable changes in blood lipid levels, which are associated with heart disease.[50]

Chocolate is another major dietary factor in promoting heart disease. The chocolate that is found in most candy bars today consists of a "compound chocolate" made of cocoa powder and vegetable fats. Many candy makers use hydrogenated soy oil, which is not at all the same as soy oil. Hydrogenated oil has had extra hydrogen ions added to change it from a liquid to a solid. Adding extra hydrogen ions to a food substance changes its chemical configuration, and we do not have the evolutionary enzymes to digest it. Hydrogenated fats, found not only in chocolate but also in margarine, cause atherosclerosis, a disorder in which cholesterol and fats are deposited on artery walls.[51]

It is, of course, next to impossible to eat chocolate without sugar, and as sugar changes the body's mineral relationships, some of these minerals become toxic. Toxic minerals cling to the cholesterol and cause hardening of the arteries. If you stay away from hydrogenated fats and sugar (which means you don't eat chocolate), effectively manage the stress in your life, and exercise regularly, you will lower your odds of developing heart disease. Research suggests it is just that easy.

WEIGHT GAIN

It may seem silly to discuss the relationship of sugar on weight gain—the connection seems so obvious. And some people may believe that they can control weight gain by simply restricting daily calorie intake. While reducing calories may, in fact, reduce weight, simply counting calories is not enough. Where did the calories come from? Carbohydrates? Fats? Protein? These are important considerations.

There is certainly a difference in the calories consumed from fresh vegetables than there is in the same number of calories from a candy bar. For one thing, when you eat calories from a sugary product, the sugar creates an artificial appetite, which causes cravings. If you give in to these cravings, you may find yourself caught in a vicious eating cycle that can lead to unnecessary weight gain and possibly obesity. Sugar overuse makes your blood sugar level yo-yo up and down, causing hunger pangs, the shakes, perspiration, and other symptoms. Sugar also causes sensitivities to certain foods, resulting in allergy-addiction. The cravings and hunger pangs that come with food allergies are certainly not conducive to dieting.

A computer is needed to calculate most diet regimes. And after all the mathematical exactitude, often the programs don't work. Calorie counting doesn't take into account how satisfied you are with what you put in your mouth. A four-ounce candy bar that is equivalent in calories to three pounds of beets or eight average-size apples doesn't go very far in satisfying an appetite. Burning the calories of a large apple requires nineteen minutes of brisk walking; burning the calories of a candy bar takes twice that. Because sugar has no vitamins, minerals, enzymes, or fiber, it satisfies neither your hunger nor your body's needs.

In a recent survey (1989–1991) of approximately 24,000 Americans, 33 percent were estimated to be overweight. Comparisons with previous surveys indicate dramatic increases in the prevalence of obesity in all races and both sexes. From 1982–1992, the prevalence of obesity increased by nearly one-third. During this period, mean body weight increased by approximately seven pounds. New data from the USDA's food consumption survey of 5,500 Americans find that people ate approximately 110 more calories per day in 1994 than they did in 1991. In 1991, people ate an average of 1,839 calories a day; in 1994, they ate 1,949. About one in three adults was considered overweight in 1994; in the 1970s, it was one in five adults.[52]

Researchers from the University of Rochester School of Medicine in New York reported that a vitamin-and-mineral-supplemented 300-calorie liquid-protein diet caused magnesium, calcium, and phosphorus depletion in the tissues of six obese patients who were on the diet for forty days. These mineral losses, which increased as the diet progressed, occurred mainly through the urine, with magnesium loss being especially great.[53] The researchers did not reveal the contents of the liquid protein, but sugar and excess protein, which commonly comprise liquid diets, can deplete minerals in the body. Liquid diets do not teach you how to eat correctly. This research also shows that such diets have a detrimental effect on the body.

We all have an internal "appestat," an appetite regulator. When we eat, our appestats tell us when we have had enough (we feel full) and we stop eating. Some people, however, have appestats that do not function properly, and they don't know when they have had enough. They can't tell when they're full, so they keep eating.

Sugar is implicated in a long chain of events in the body that leads to weight gain. The minerals in the body become unbalanced, enzymes don't function correctly, food does not digest properly, and allergies occur. Allergies cause addiction, addiction causes cravings, and overeating is the result. So forget simple calorie counting. If you want to lose some pounds or keep from gaining unnecessary weight, eliminate sugar and other refined foods—such as white flour, spaghetti, and pizza—from your diet. Get back to the basics: exercise regularly and eat meals that include lots of vegetables, legumes, protein, and grains.

PREMENSTRUAL SYNDROME

Premenstrual syndrome (PMS) is characterized by a combination of mental and physical complaints that arise sometimes up to a week before a woman gets her menstrual period. PMS can occur without personality instability or neurosis, although there has been a correlation between severity of neurosis and the intensity of PMS symptoms.[54] These symptoms commonly include cravings, cramps, headaches, bloating, water retention, insomnia, weight gain, depression, anxiety, irritability, anger, and mood swings.

There are many food items that can cause PMS symptoms. Sugar binges in PMS women have been noted.[55] Researchers at Oregon State University sent a questionnaire to its female students. The survey regarded menstrual and premenstrual health in conjunction with daily dietary practices. The consumption of chocolate, which cannot be eaten without a lot of sugar, alcoholic beverages, fruit juice, and caffeine-free cola was prevalent in those with the most severe symptoms.[56]

Today's glamorous American female—long-legged and ultra-lean—represents a developmental deficit, not a plus. This body development reveals an imbalance between growth hormone and inefficient production of female hormones brought about by dietary factors over generations. Those with anorexia nervosa are extreme examples of this hormone imbalance. As the patients get thinner and thinner their menstrual cycles cease.[57]

Symptoms of PMS are caused by the same upset body chemistry that causes other symptoms. This chemical imbalance prevents glands from secreting the necessary amount of hormones; for some, this insufficiency causes PMS. If you experience uncomfortable premenstrual symptoms, work on maintaining a well-balanced lifestyle. Eat right, exercise, and deal with the distress in your life (see the four "arenas" beginning on page 155). Eat only those foods listed in Food Plan III (page 163). I also suggest dividing your three meals into six smaller ones, so you have something in your stomach much of the day. Test for homeostasis, as discussed Chapter 9. When you find yourself in homeostasis for two menstrual cycles, those uncomfortable symptoms will likely be gone.

CANDIDIASIS

Candida albicans is a yeastlike fungus that inhabits the gastrointestinal tract, the genitourinary tract, the mouth, the esophagus, and the throat. All people, babies and adults alike, have this organism, which normally lives in healthy balance with the other bacteria in the body. Certain conditions may cause the candida to multiply, causing an infection known as candidiasis.[58]

When the body is out of homeostasis and there are only six or so functioning units of calcium in the bloodstream rather than the usual ten, the cells become deficient and inefficient. The immune system is weakened and cannot handle the candida, which begins to grow uncontrollably. Diets rich in sugar can stimulate the fungal growth, as can birth control pills, cortisone and cortisonelike drugs, antibiotics, and immunosuppressant drugs used in cancer therapy and other therapies. These drugs kill off the good bacteria and leave space for the fungus to proliferate.

Dr. C. Orion Truss, the grandfather of candidiasis research, discovered that when candida overgrows, it secretes an estrogen very much like the body's own estrogen. In fact, this estrogen can substitute for the body's estrogen. Candida's estrogen can occupy the binding sites of our cells and prevent regular estrogen from getting in. Unfortunately, candida's estrogen is only $\frac{1}{100}$ as potent as the estrogen that is normally produced by the body. If all the binding sites where regular estrogen is needed are filled with something that is only $\frac{1}{100}$ as potent, and you are already estrogen-starved, you are in trouble.[59,60]

When candidiasis affects the mouth it is called thrush. White sores may form on the tongue, gums, and inside the cheeks. Candida overgrowth in the geritourinary tract may result in kidney and bladder infections, or vaginitis, which is characterized by intense vaginal burning and itching and a white cheesy discharge. In the gastrointestinal tract, common symptoms of candidiasis are indigestion, bloating, diarrhea or constipation, fatigue, gas, and allergic reactions.[61]

Candida overgrowth can cause other troubles as well. When *Candida albicans*, which is normally round, starts to overgrow in the intestines, it enters the mycelia stage and grows roots that penetrate the intestinal walls. Once the candida is overgrown, the tissue integrity of the wall is compromised, and the wall becomes very weak. If you kill the root at this time through antifungal drugs or other aids, you risk leaving a hole in the intestinal wall through which undigested food can pass. The immune system will be unable to handle the food, and you will become allergic to it.[62] As the body heals, so will the intestinal wall.

We may think of ourselves as victims of this fungus,

but we are not. We have to feed the candida in order for it to grow. And as sugar is the main substance that feeds candida, the elimination of sugar from the diet is one effective cure. But candida also loves wine and all other alcoholic beverages, as well as yeast, mushrooms, aged cheese, nuts, seeds, and fruits. Food Plan III (see page 163) is the best diet for those with candidiasis. And since distress also upsets the body and suppresses the immune system, learning to deal with life's daily stresses is another important factor in maintaining a healthy balance of *Candida albicans*.[63]

TOOTH DECAY

The secretion of excess calcium is one clear sign of a mineral imbalance; tooth decay is another. Many clinicians believe that the first sign of any degenerative disease process is seen in the mouth. If you had many cavities as a child, chances are you will have many diseases as an adult—unless you maintain a proper balance in your body chemistry.

Almost every tooth in my mouth has a gold, silver (amalgam), or composite filling. When I was a teenager, my parents had the dentist replace all of my amalgam fillings with gold. For about four months I went to the dentist every Monday to have this work done. My dentist didn't believe in painkillers; whenever he was near a nerve, my pain would let him know. I can still vividly remember dreading those Mondays.

Then, as an adult—until I stopped eating sugar—I had to go to the dentist every three months rather than the usual six because so much plaque would build on my teeth. Between visits, I would scrape the back of my teeth with a nail pick to remove the plaque. Now that sugar is out of my diet, I see the dentist only once every six months, and my teeth have little or no plaque.

Studies have shown a definite correlation between tooth decay and the amounts of calcium, magnesium, and phosphorus in the body. When the levels of these minerals in one study group were examined, the group with two or more dental cavities per year was found to have higher than normal calcium and magnesium levels in the blood, but lower than normal phosphorus levels, particularly in the saliva. In this same study, 10 percent of those tested had adequate phosphorus levels in their saliva. This was reflected in a finding of one cavity or less per person, and most of the people in this category had no decay at all.[64]

When the phosphorus level drops or increases due to the ingestion of sugar, and the calcium-phosphorus ratio becomes unbalanced, an acid state occurs in the mouth. Acid is also formed when the bacteria in the tooth plaque interact with sugar. A pH scale, which ranges from 1 to 14, is used to determine the acidity or alkalinity of a solution. The value of 7.0 is neutral; below 7.0 is acidic; above 7.0 is alkaline. Tooth enamel begins to dissolve when the saliva is around pH 5.5. After the ingestion of sugar, the pH value on the surface of the teeth may drop as low as 4.5 and remain low for about twenty minutes before slowly returning to a neutral state. And this return from an acid state to a normal one occurs only if the saliva has adequate minerals to do so. The repeated consumption of sugar causes a continual production of acid in the mouth. As with osteoporosis, it is clear that removing sugar and other substances that cause a calcium-phosphorus imbalance is a necessary step in stopping this degenerative process.

Dentists tell us to brush and floss often, and to keep

babies from falling asleep with juice- or milk-filled bottles in their mouths. These suggestions, while certainly helpful in maintaining good oral health, presume that if sugar is not allowed to linger in the mouth, there is no danger of tooth decay. Keeping the body in homeostasis, however, is most critical. Anything that affects the teeth can't help but affect the rest of the body, and imbalances plaguing the body will affect the teeth as well.

When you are in homeostasis, your teeth secrete mucus microscopically. It is how the teeth cleanse themselves. Cells within the pulp tissue of the teeth do the secreting and cleansing; the secretion comes through the enamel rods of the teeth and keeps them from decaying. When you are not in homeostasis, when you have eaten sugar, for example, this microscopic cleansing system does not work effectively; something quite different happens.

Ralph Steinman, a researcher from Loma Linda University, put feeding tubes down the throats of rats to bypass their teeth. He then fed the rats sugar water through the tubes. Within a matter of minutes, the fluid movement of the tooth secretion reversed. Instead of the cleansing fluids moving from the inner pulp of the teeth to the outer enamel, the fluids in the mouth began penetrating the enamel rods, making their way into the dentin. The bacterial by-products in the mouth are acidic; and as long as this fluid movement comes from within the teeth, the acid won't decalcify the enamel. But when this normal process is reversed, and mouth fluids start entering the teeth from the outside, decalcification begins. This suggests, at least in part, that tooth decay is due to a system malfunction, and not just a tooth-surface problem.[65]

While it's true that the ingestion of sugar starts in the

mouth, and that is where tooth decay occurs, this study seems to show that decay comes from an unbalanced body chemistry. Unless the body is thought of as a whole, rather than a number of parts, the truly deleterious effects of sugar cannot be fully measured.

MULTIPLE SCLEROSIS

Multiple sclerosis (MS) is a progressive, degenerative disease of the central nervous system. MS is widely believed to be an autoimmune disease in which the white blood cells attack the myelin sheaths that cover the nerves. Although the cause of MS is not known, one popular theory is that it is caused by food intolerances or allergic reactions. I call it an allergy of the nervous system.

In a controlled study of 135 multiple sclerosis patients, it was found that of these subjects, 65.9 percent had histories of sinusitis. This inflammation of the sinuses is a classic allergy symptom that is often linked to dairy products. The removal of dairy products from the patients' diets resulted in the disappearance of the sinusitis as well as a number of other MS symptoms.[66]

Clinician and researcher Arthur Kaslow, M.D. found that many foods caused symptoms of MS. Overcooked red meat, sugar, fruits, and flour products were frequent culprits. Yet different foods affected people differently. Dr. Kaslow also found that some foods that were tolerated in small quantities were not well-tolerated in large quantities. Large amounts of any food cannot be tolerated by people with upset body chemistry. He concluded that small amounts of food eaten five or six times a day, less any foods to which the patient has an allergic reaction, is the best diet.[67] I couldn't agree more. Food Plan III (see page 163) is recommended for those who have MS.

INFLAMMATORY BOWEL DISEASE

Inflammatory bowel disease has two major categories. One is ulcerative colitis, which affects the inner lining of the colon. The other is Crohn's disease, which can irritate the deeper layers of the intestinal wall.

Any segment of the intestinal wall—twenty feet of small intestine and five feet of large intestine—is vulnerable to inflammatory bowel disease. Depending on the area affected, this disease is known by many other names: regional enteritis, ileitis, colitis, granulomatous colitis, and ileo colitis.[68]

Usual symptoms are diarrhea, weight loss, and cramping. Yet blood, urine, and stool tests, as well as barium enemas may show the bowel to be normal. Some patients display other symptoms not associated with the gastrointestinal tract such as hay fever, headaches, asthma, arthritis, and fatigue.

A variety of studies have shown that most people with inflammatory bowel disease can control their symptoms by eliminating foods to which they react. Although any food can cause symptoms, those that most commonly cause problems are sugar, wheat, milk, corn, coffee, tea, and citrus fruits.[69]

The best way to determine the abusive foods is to withdraw all foods for twelve hours or until the symptoms have stopped. Then introduce one food at a time and watch for symptoms. Research from various sources shows that people who suffer from inflammatory bowel disease can live symptom-free once they have eliminated the problem-causing food or foods.

It is wise for people with inflammatory bowel disease to introduce acidophilus into their diets. Acidophilus will help maintain a balance of healthy bacteria in the gastrointestinal tract. Effective stress management is another important strategy in minimizing the symptoms.

CANKER SORES (APTHOUS ULCERS)

Painful canker sores, which occur in the mouth, can appear on the tongue, on the insides of the cheeks, on the lips, or on the gums. The sores can be as small as a pinhead or as large as a quarter. They are often preceded by a burning and tingling sensation, which is followed by the appearance of painful red spots in the mouth. Unlike fever blisters, canker sores do not form blisters. They appear quickly and generally take from four to twenty days to heal.[70]

Canker sores may be triggered by a number of factors—stress and food allergies being the most common culprits. Studies done in Australia indicate that the incidence of canker sores can be stopped with the elimination of offending foods from the diet. Patients with recurring canker sores of the tongue and mouth were unresponsive to medications over a period of months. Twelve of these patients were then placed on a restricted diet for eight weeks. Half of the people had complete clearing of the sores, which promptly recurred with food challenge. The offending foods identified in the study were dairy products, wheat, chocolate, tomato products, vinegar, citrus, and pineapple.[71]

The study did not specify whether or not the subjects were allowed to eat sugar or other offending foods, which could have further upset their body chemistry, making them allergic to other foods. I believe that if *all* abusive foods had been removed from their diets, all twelve subjects would have responded to treatment.

GALLSTONES

The gallbladder is a small sac-like organ that lies under the liver. It receives, stores, and concentrates the bile that is made in the liver. During digestion, the gallbladder sends the bile to the intestines to help break down the fat that is contained in food.

Gallstones—mineral deposits consisting of bile pigments and calcium salts—are a common problem associated with the gallbladder. Gallstones may cause inflammation and blockage of the gallbladder, and abdominal pain (usually right-sided).[72] Other symptoms might include bloating, belching, and intolerance to foods.[73] Right-sided shoulder pain may also occur.

One of every ten Americans has gallstones. This risk increases to one of every five after age forty. Gallstones may go unnoticed or they may cause pain—wrenching pain.[74]

A recent article in the *British Medical Journal*, entitled "The Sweet Road to Gallstones," reported that refined sugar may be one of the major dietary risk factors in gallstone formation. Sugar and other abusive foods can upset the body's minerals. When such an imbalance causes calcium to become toxic or nonfunctioning, the calcium can deposit itself anywhere in the body, including the gallbladder.[75]

KIDNEY STONES

Kidney stones, which form when mineral salts clump together in the urine, are composed mainly of calcium and/or phosphorus. Stones may form anywhere in the entire urinary tract—the kidneys, the bladder, and the urinary ducts. Depending on the stone's size and location,

symptoms range from severe pain to no pain at all.
Commonly, kidney stones cause severe, excruciating
back pain that comes on suddenly. This pain may be
associated with nausea and vomiting, abdominal bloating, blood in the urine, pain upon urination, chills, and
fever.

High levels of sugar in the diet may encourage stone
formation, as sugar stimulates the pancreas to release
insulin, which stimulates calcium excretion through
the urine.[76] Chronic dehydration may also increase the
possibility of kidney stone formation.[77] Increased dietary levels of soft drinks, coffee, protein, and salt are
also suspect.[78]

Go back to basics. Work on getting and keeping your
body in homeostasis. Refer to Chapter 9 for positive
lifestyle guidelines. Follow the food plans and work on
managing the distress in your life.

CYSTIC FIBROSIS

Cystic fibrosis is a hereditary disease that mainly affects
the pancreas, respiratory system, and sweat glands.
Symptoms of cystic fibrosis begin early in life. Glands
in the lungs and bronchial tubes secrete thick mucus that
blocks lung passages and traps harmful bacteria, resulting in chronic respiratory problems. Thick secretions
also often obstruct the release of pancreatic enzymes, resulting in digestive difficulties and malabsorption problems. Malnutrition may result because a lack of necessary
digestive enzymes means nutrients from foods—particularly selenium and zinc—are not properly absorbed. Once
a person becomes deficient in one mineral, then the functioning of the other minerals becomes impaired also.[79]

Dr. Joel Wallach has been improving the health of

cystic fibrosis patients by eliminating reactive foods from their diets. This gives the small intestine a chance to heal itself and allows increased absorption of selenium, zinc, protein, essential fatty acids, and other nutrients. This, in turn, allows the mineral-dependent pancreatic enzymes to function more readily, enabling food to digest properly.[80]

Because the person with cystic fibrosis has a pancreas that doesn't function optimally, it is very important for this person to maintain a balanced body chemistry. Keeping this balance is one way to help achieve an acceptable level of wellness.

FUTURE GENERATIONS

Changing your dietary habits can do more than help you avoid causing ailments like those listed here. And if you are of childbearing age or younger, you have a chance to improve the expression of the genetic blueprint of your children.

All of us, from time to time, have noticed things about ourselves that are inherited from our parents—the color of our eyes, the shape of our nose, certain personality traits, and so on. We also inherit genetic strengths and weaknesses, particularly in the glands of the endocrine system, which can have a healthy expression or an unhealthy one, depending on the condition of one's body chemistry (see the Four Arenas beginning on page 155). If we abuse our bodies over and over with sugar and other harmful substances, these inherited strengths and weaknesses can express ill health and eventually degenerative disease processes may result. Even worse, the weak expression we create in our bodies may be expressed in our children as well.

When continual lifestyle abuse causes an unbalanced body chemistry, the resulting weak expression of one's endocrine system can be passed down and magnified over generations with increasingly serious consequences. Conversely, when any individual, through informed action, continuously allows harmonious body chemistry, he or she will enjoy better health, and the offspring will exhibit a better expression of the genetic blueprint than the parents.

Francis Pottenger studied cats over several generations. He fed one group of cats a primitive diet of raw foods; a second group received the same foods, only cooked; and a third group was given the cooked-food diet accompanied by condensed milk, which contains sugar. The cats in the first group lived the longest and gave birth to healthy cats over several generations. The second group of cats did not live as long as those in the first group and gave birth to two generations of cats, each of which was less healthy than the former generation. Although the cats in both of these groups ate the same food, cooking appeared to alter some of the nutrient availability.

Adding sugar to this cooked-food diet made these nutrients even less available, as shown by the deterioration over three generations of the third group of cats. These cats, who drank the condensed milk, gave birth to second and third generations with many abnormalities, including hair that was not as shiny and thick as in the first generation. When kept on the cooked, sweetened food, the third generation was not able to reproduce. Interestingly, when these third-generation cats were switched to an all raw-food diet, they became healthy enough to reproduce and give birth to kittens who were healthier than those of the third generation.

This demonstrates that the potential expression in the genetic blueprint is inhibited by lifestyle. Like these cats, each of us inherits an endocrine pattern from our parents and we pass this pattern on to our children. Our lifestyles determine how our genetic expressions are manifested—healthy or unhealthy.[81]

A few years ago, I took a trip to Egypt. Although most of the people would not be considered middle class by our standards, no one is starving. The Egyptian government subsidizes a healthful whole wheat bread, which we call pita bread. In many villages along the Nile, I observed primitive methods for making this bread, which consists solely of whole wheat flour and water. A twelve-inch-round pita costs one cent, so it is easily affordable and available to everyone.

The hotels I stayed in, however, served breakfasts that included white-bread toast, croissants, and white-flour rolls with jelly. Even when I asked for Egyptian bread at the hotels, most of the time I couldn't get it. On the streets I saw the people eating breakfasts of falafel (chick pea-and-bean-stuffed pita bread) or pita bread stuffed with okra, lettuce, tomato, and small amounts of beef. In the hotels, where the clientele was more affluent, refined foods prevailed. When I returned to Cairo, what little pita bread I saw was made of white flour and was very expensive. White flour, not whole wheat, was used in the bakeries of Cairo to make breads, cakes, and pastries.

The living conditions are still primitive in many Egyptian villages. The sanitary conditions are poor, and I'm sure that there are many deaths at birth and during infancy due to unsanitary conditions and communicable diseases. No doubt such living conditions will improve in the years to come, life expectancy will increase, and the favorite foods of the so-called advanced nations, sugar and white flour, will become more and more popular. As a result, the quality of the added years will undoubtedly be marred by arthritis, osteoporosis, cancer, heart disease, and other degenerative diseases. The endocrine systems of the villagers will start to wear down, and the weaknesses will be passed on to future generations. Affluence seems synonymous with refined foods, cakes, pastries, tobacco, and other abusive substances. The more affluent people become, the further they stray from their native diet, and the weaker they and future generations become.

There is no way to change your endocrine blueprint once you become an adult, but a healthy, well-balanced lifestyle can make a difference in the way you feel now and in the future. The continual use of sugar and other abusive foods, or the use of foods to which you are allergic depletes the ability of the endocrine gland to function properly. When these glands are abused day in and day out, over a period of years and eventually through several generations, a certain degree of nonfunctioning and abnormal functioning of these overworked glands occurs.

CONCLUSION

It is interesting to note that in spite of the incredible sums of money and research hours spent on investigating diseases, overall, disease in the United States is increasing. The exception is cardiovascular disease, which has decreased, not due to any medicines, but rather to lifestyle changes—exercise, stress reduction, and healthy eating habits. Diseases and conditions such as cancer, diabetes, epilepsy, migraine headaches, chronic sinusitis and bronchitis, and allergies are on the rise. Diabetes is on a significant rise.

Any disease state is the body's way of protesting an abusive lifestyle. I don't know why life needs to be so confusing when it seems so easy. Just take away from the body what it doesn't need and give it what it does need to keep it healthy. In the next chapter, we'll examine other substances—including alcohol, caffeine, and food additives—which, like sugar, must be avoided for a body to maintain a healthy balance.

6
Sugar's Helpers

B y now, it should be obvious that eliminating sugar from your diet is an essential step in keeping healthy and avoiding degenerative disease. Simply going without sugar is not enough. There are many other harmful substances such as alcohol, caffeine, rancid fats, aspirin, artificial sweeteners, mercury and other toxic metals, and food additives that should be avoided in order to maintain good health.

ALCOHOL

Alcohol, like sugar, is absorbed very quickly into the bloodstream. The absorption process begins in the mouth and continues in the esophagus and stomach. Because alcoholic beverages are made from various grains (wheat, rye, corn, and barley), the residue from these grains also moves quickly into the bloodstream. Many people who drink alcoholic beverages regularly or excessively can become allergic to these grains. The repeated exposure to alcohol can exhaust the enzymes necessary to digest these residues. As discussed in Chapter 2, this exhaustion causes undigested food to be absorbed into the bloodstream, resulting in allergies.

Alcohol that is not absorbed quickly reaches the large intestine and expands the cells of the intestinal lining.[1] The alcohol and any other food that happens to be in the intestine can also be absorbed into the bloodstream without being completely digested. When alcohol is consumed with meals, then, there is a four times greater risk of allergic reaction than there is when drinking alcohol alone.[2] Alcohol has the same effect on the body as sugar—and if you're drinking alcohol with added sugar (found in many mixed drinks and cocktails), you are subjecting your body to a doubly harmful dose.

Dr. George Ulett, director of Neuropsychiatric Service and Psychosomatic Research Lab of Deaconess Hospital in St. Louis, tested three groups of people—social drinkers, members of Alcoholics Anonymous (AA), and active alcoholics—to see which group had the most food allergies. He found that the active alcoholics were, as suspected, reactive to more foods than those in the other two groups. Social drinkers were next, and the members of AA, who consumed no alcohol at all, had the least number of food allergies. It seems obvious that alcohol is detrimental to the body's ability to digest and assimilate food properly.[3] It is, therefore, wise to limit your alcohol consumption.

When alcohol upsets the body chemistry, the digestive system suffers. Jean Poulos and Donald Stoddard's research shows a correlation between alcohol and blood sugar problems. Through their studies, they discovered that 100 percent of the alcoholics involved in their research were either hypoglycemic, pre-diabetic, or diabetic.[4]

During interviews conducted at various Alcoholics Anonymous meetings, I asked members the following question: "Do you remember eating a lot of sugar as a child?" Many recalled eating sugar and sugar-laden foods obsessively as part of their daily childhood routine. Some did not remember eating a lot of sugar-sweetened candies and baked goods, but did recall drinking as many as five or six soft drinks a day. One person even recounted a habit of eating sugar straight from the sugar bowl. The idea that alcoholics are former sugarholics has been verified by Graham Golditz, who found that the consumption of candy and sugar is inversely related to alcohol intake. He discovered that sugar craving decreases when alcohol is consumed. However, when alcohol consumption stops, sugar intake increases.[5]

Not all people who are sugarholics as children will grow up to be alcoholics, but there does seem to be a correlation between sugar addiction and alcohol addiction. Alcoholics Anonymous helps recovering alcoholics tremendously by providing psychological and educational support. It is ironic that coffee, donuts, and other sugar-sweetened foods are provided at the meetings. These foods can further suppress the immune system of those who are already nutritionally deficient (such as most alcoholics).[6] Sugar can lower the blood sugar level and put these people in a hypoglycemic state—with all the symptoms of withdrawal and cravings for alcohol.

When alcohol is in the stomach or small intestine, food does not digest as quickly. It was reported at a science symposium that a larger amount of food was retained in the stomach following alcohol intake as compared when no alcohol was consumed. The longer food stays in the stomach, the harder the body must work to digest it.

Studies also show that alcohol changes the body's

ability to metabolize zinc. A person might be getting enough zinc in his or her diet, but if alcohol is also consumed, the cells are less capable of utilizing that zinc, and a deficiency results. This deficiency is considered the principal cause of cirrhosis of the liver, a disease characterized by progressive destruction of liver cells and liver shrinkage. When even moderate amounts of alcohol are ingested, there is an immediate decrease of zinc in the liver. As little as four alcoholic beverages a day over a period of time can cause liver damage.[7]

As the majority of alcoholics get most of their calories from alcohol, rather than nutritious foods, they are more than likely to have a nutrient deficiency. In addition, food absorbed too quickly through the alcohol-expanded walls of the small intestine cannot provide the body with nutrients. The intestinal mucosa doesn't have time to absorb vitamins and minerals.[8] And it can take from months to years to recover these normal physiological capacities. Eating four or five small meals daily that include protein, complex carbohydrates, and some fats, supplemented with vitamins and minerals, is a positive step toward helping heal an unbalanced body that has been abused by alcohol.

The link between sugar and alcohol is vividly seen in an experiment conducted by Dr. Ruth Adams. Dr. Adams put laboratory rats on a nutrient-deficient diet of coffee, donuts, hot dogs, soft drinks, apple pie, spaghetti and meatballs, canned green beans, white bread, and cake—primarily foods with hidden and not-so-hidden sugar. Eighty percent of the rats on this diet preferred to drink alcohol instead of water. In fact, they had a craving for alcohol. The other 20 percent preferred water that had been sugar sweetened. When half of the rats were put back on a healthful diet, their alcohol consumption dropped. The rats who stayed on the poor diet continued to increase their alcohol consumption.[9]

A recent study indicated that sugar, white flour, and refined carbohydrates are addictive substances that have similar effects on brain neurotransmitters as alcohol. Trying to go "cold turkey" from a steady diet of these foods can result in withdrawal symptoms like headaches, dizziness, and depression. Current research indicates that sugar and refined carbohydrates increase brain production of the chemicals dopamine, serotonin, and norepinephrine. This leads to a "high" that is similar to the type induced by alcohol and other drugs. Thus, the researchers advise those suffering from alcoholism to give up sugar and products made from white flour. Clearly, sugar increases the craving for alcohol, and alcohol promotes the same kind of bodily harm as sugar.

Physiological withdrawal symptoms from alcohol are usually gone within ten days. Unfortunately, during stressful times, people may have cravings for alcohol and refined carbohydrates. Although these cravings are more psychological than physical, they are still very real. It is important to identify what is causing your cravings, rather than trying to "fix" them. I do not think that "candy is dandy" or "liquor is quicker." Sorry, Ogden Nash.

CAFFEINE

Caffeine is a slightly bitter alkaloid that is found in and commonly associated with coffee and tea. It is also found in cola nuts and cocoa, which accounts for its presence in a variety of soft drinks and chocolate products.

A stimulant, caffeine can actually increase the amount of sugar in the bloodstream. When ingested, caffeine stimulates the adrenal glands, which release adrenaline-like substances called *catecholamines*. These catecholamines cause the heart to pump harder than normal and the liver to release stored sugar, which raises the blood sugar level.[10] In turn, the pancreas secretes insulin to bring the level down to normal. This process, as explained in Chapter 4, can result in the eventual exhaustion of the pancreas.

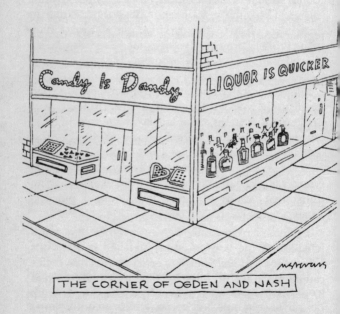

THE CORNER OF OGDEN AND NASH

Drawing by M. Stevens; © 1996 The New Yorker Magazine, Inc.

This release of sugar causes the "lift" most people associate with caffeine, but because caffeine also throws the body chemistry out of balance, the lift is short-lived. The rush of insulin from the pancreas frequently goes so far beyond restoring normality that the sugar level falls below normal, causing extreme fatigue and other hypoglycemic symptoms. It may be hours before the body's chemistry returns to normal, and if another cup of coffee or tea has been ingested, the cycle of imbalance will continue.[11]

Caffeine is implicated in a number of other problems as well. There is a possible connection between caffeine intake and birth defects, benign breast lumps, and irregular heartbeat. As caffeine stimulates the central nervous system, it has also been linked to insomnia, nervousness, and anxiety. It is also a cardiac muscle stimulant, a diuretic, and a stimulant of gastric acid secretion in the stomach. In 1980, the FDA advised pregnant women to avoid or minimize the consumption of products containing caffeine.[12]

Noted biochemist Jeffrey Bland, Ph.D., can't say enough nasty things about coffee. His studies show, among other things, that caffeine elevates cholesterol levels in the blood. Bland also explains that the reason for the frequency of ulcers in coffee drinkers is that coffee stimulates the secretion of gastric juices.[13]

Caffeine isn't the only element in coffee that plays havoc with the body. A study detailed in the Tufts University *Diet and Nutrition Letter* shows that coffee can inhibit iron absorption by 39 percent, or as much as 87 percent when coffee or tea is consumed with or up to one hour after a meal. (Drinking coffee or tea before the meal did not have the same effect.) One of the authors of the study, Dr. James D. Cook, claims that it it isn't the caffeine that interferes with iron absorption but a family of binding substances called polyphenols (tannic acid), which are found in coffee and tea. This group of chemicals strong-arms iron and escorts it out of the body. Since decaffeinated coffee also contains polyphenols, it too carries off needed iron.[14] Herbal tea, which is not believed to prevent iron absorption, is a good alternative for those who want to give up coffee and regular forms of tea.

In spite of caffeine's implication in heart disease, gastritis, heartburn, calcium secretion, increased stomach acid and stomach discomfort, cystic breast conditions, and nervousness and anxiety, the public continues to consume mountains of coffee beans, tea leaves, and cacao nuts. Dr. Eyi Takaahushi, of the Tohoku University School of Medicine, has found a correlation between the amount of coffee a country consumes and the number of deaths from cancer of the prostate. Other data indicate that it is the sugar used in coffee, rather than the coffee itself, that is the cause of prostate cancer. A definite correlation was also found between sugar consumption and cancer of the breast, ovaries, intestine, and rectum.[15] (More good reasons to switch from caffeinated beverages to herbal tea.)

DRUGS

Drug use causes an imbalance in the body chemistry. All drugs must be detoxified or undergo some change within the body before they can be eliminated. This detoxification usually takes place in the liver with the aid of enzymes, which are mineral-dependent. Drug overuse or abuse causes a continually upset chemical balance, resulting in the eventual exhaustion of the enzymes and minerals necessary for the detoxification process.

Certain drugs can add an extra burden to an already compromised body. For example, antacids, in addition to damaging the digestive system, can cause mineral imbalances that result in bone damage. Cortisone raises the blood sugar to higher than normal levels. My research with urine calcium secretion shows that many antibiotics increase the presence of calcium in the urine, thereby upsetting the body chemistry. Let's take a closer look at some of these drugs.

Antacids

Most antacids, generally taken for the relief of heartburn and indigestion, contain aluminum chloride. (One exception is Tums.) Antacids that contain aluminum, such as the popular stomach medications Mylanta and Maalox, in addition to damaging the digestive tract, cause a mineral imbalance.

These aluminum-containing antacids work by binding with and neutralizing gastric acid. Unfortunately, they also prevent the absorption of phosphoric acid, which is then eliminated in the stool. To compensate for this loss of phosphorus, the bones release some of their phosphorus into the bloodstream, along with the calcium to which it was bound. This calcium is quickly carried away by the kidneys and eliminated through the urine.[16]

Aluminum-containing antacids, taken year after year, can deplete the bones of their much-needed calcium and phosphorus, resulting in bone thinning and weakness. Minor activities such as bending over to tie one's shoes and walking up stairs can lead to bone fractures—a condition in which the bones crack but do not break completely. The resulting stiffness, weakness, and pain are often mistaken for arthritis. Unfortunately, it takes years for the cumulative negative effects of repeated antacid use to materialize. Sadly, at this stage in life, people tend to accept bone pain and fractures as a natural part of aging.[17]

Antacids—with or without aluminum—also harm the bones by interfering with digestion. Calcium is absorbed in the upper part of the small intestine, and hydrochloric acid is essential for the digestive process. Most antacids are used by people over forty years old, whose normal amount of hydrochloric acid has already decreased along with their calcium absorption. Antacids are generally taken for heartburn and "overly acidic" stomachs. Chances are the stomach is actually secreting *less* hydrochloric acid than is necessary for proper digestion.

The simplest and most effective way to deal with heartburn and indigestion is to prevent such conditions from happening in the first place. For instance, eliminate caffeine from your diet; it stimulates the secretion of gastric juices. Don't overeat at any one meal; it exhausts the necessary digestive juices. And remove all sugar from your diet; it has been shown time and time again to throw off the body's chemical balance. Dr. John Yudkin has studied acidity and digestive activity before and after sugar ingestion in healthy people. The results show that just two weeks of a sugar-rich diet is long enough to increase both stomach acidity and digestive activity of gastric juices—found in those with gastric or duodenal ulcers. The sugar increased stomach acidity by approximately 20 percent, and the enzyme activity tripled.

Antibiotics

There is no arguing the fact that antibiotics are useful in the treatment of certain infections. Today, however, antibiotics are frequently overused. We live in a society in which we demand "quick fixes" for our maladies. Commonly, doctors overprescribe antibiotics rather than allow the body to heal itself.

Common side effects from antibiotics include rashes, fever, bronchial tube spasms, blood vessel inflammation, kidney and ear problems, upset stomach, vomiting, fatigue, and insomnia.[18] Overuse of antibiotics can result in the following more-serious adverse affects:

- *Suppression of the immune system.* A flow of studies on the use of antibiotics and the immune system have been conducted since the 1950s. Most researchers agree that antibiotics display a suppression of antibody (immune fighter) production and impairment of phagocytosis (process by which foreign invaders are gobbled up) by the white blood cells.

- *Reduction of potentially helpful bacteria.*

- *Promotion of antibiotic-resistant microorganisms.*

- *Invasive overgrowth of yeast, resulting in a Candida-related syndrome.*[19] (See additional information on candidiasis beginning on page 95.)

When used prudently, antibiotics can, indeed, be effective in fighting a number of bacterial infections. Be careful, however, not to rush to take antibiotics for that "quick fix." When possible, allow your body's natural defenses to do the job.

Aspirin

Although aspirin is not a food, many people take it regularly. Doctors prescribe it for everything from headaches and menstrual problems to joint pains and heart disease. Indeed, there is evidence of aspirin's positive effects.

One researcher found high levels of prostaglandins (potent hormone-like chemicals that aid in the formation of blood clots; high levels are implicated in heart disease) in infected chickens. When these chickens were fed aspirin, the prostaglandin levels dropped and the mortality rate fell from 80 percent to 42 percent in two days. The aspirin clearly blocked the prostaglandins and improved the resistance to infection.[20]

Yet agents such as aspirin, which inhibit one or more of the enzymes involved in prostaglandin synthesis, may cause negative alterations of body function. Researcher Dr. Edith Stanley found that aspirin blocked an area of the immune system needed for the healing process. Aspirin kept the infection-fighting leukocytes from traveling to the inflammatory tissue. By suppressing the body's natural response to infection, aspirin may "relieve" the symptoms caused by the leukocytes battling the invading virus, but the reproduction of the virus is left unchecked. If leukocytes continue to be hindered, the virus is then free to spread within the body, prolonging and complicating the illness.[21]

Leukocytes are not the only blood components adversely affected by aspirin; platelets—those cells in the blood that are necessary for clotting—are also disrupted. When a blood vessel ruptures, collagen tissue, which makes up the basement membrane of blood vessels, is exposed. The collagen signals the platelets to release a mineral substance, adenosine diphosphate, which makes the platelets sticky enough to bind together. Aspirin can destroy adenosine diphosphate, making the platelets incapable of binding to one another. As few as one or two 350-mg aspirin tablets can have this negative effect on the blood platelets, which remain in this condition for about seven days—the life span of each individual platelet. One 350-mg dose of aspirin, then, can permanently destroy a platelet's ability to clump together with other platelets when necessary. Anyone who takes two 350-mg aspirins twice a day is maintaining a consistently ineffective platelet system and cutting down on the body's normal response to external injury.[22]

In one study, Dr. Stanley gave aspirin to a group of people who were sick with a viral infection. Another group who also had a viral infection received a placebo. Dr. Stanley discovered that the group treated with aspirin had a 17 to 30 percent increase in viruses. Also, the nasal discharge of those treated with aspirin was considerably greater than that of the untreated group. And interestingly, the average illness length was longer in the treated group.[23] Another researcher, Dr. N.M.H. Graham from Johns Hopkins School of Hygiene and Public Health, found that in a study of patients with viral infections, there was a suppression of the immune system in those given aspirin.[24]

Researchers have found that aspirin and other pain medications can cause irreversible damage to the kidneys and lead to kidney failure. It doesn't take very much. Just three 350-mg aspirin a day (two kilograms in six years) can seriously impair the vital cleansing function of the kidneys. For those people living in hot climates or those on low-salt diets the problem is even more serious.[25] A group of British researchers found that a daily aspirin dose of 1500 milligrams (approximately four aspirins) caused a significant incidence in upper gastrointestinal bleeding, peptic ulcers, and other gastrointestinal upsets.[26]

I wish that I could report that other analgesics such as acetaminophen (Tylenol) and ibuprofen (Advil) are good substitutes for aspirin, but I cannot. Current research indicates that these drugs are also associated with gastrointestinal upset, headaches, and dizziness.[27]

A recent study has linked the use of aspirin by children and teenagers to Reye's syndrome. Fatal in 20 to 30 percent of the cases, Reye's syndrome begins with a sudden onset of vomiting, often with fever and sometimes accompanied by lethargy, severe headaches, and changes in behavior. These symptoms can progress quickly to convulsions, delirium, and coma. Another study, conducted by the Centers for Disease Control, found that children suffering from the flu or chicken pox were twelve to twenty-five times more likely to develop Reye's syndrome when given aspirin.[28]

It is aspirin's destruction of the intestinal lining that is most important in the link between food allergies and the immune system. When the intestinal lining is damaged, large food molecules are able to pass through, allowing undigested protein to enter the bloodstream. This can cause an allergic reaction and immune response.

Like sugar and alcohol, aspirin can be a direct cause of food allergies.[29] All in all, it is better to let the natural healing process progress on its own, without the help of aspirin.

Other Drug Dangers

Pharmaceutical drugs, both prescription and over-the-counter, have side effects that are mild to serious in nature. All cause some type of chemical imbalance.

For example, thiazide diuretics, which are taken to alleviate fluid retention, can deplete magnesium and cause leg cramps and general weakness. And as these drugs can cause abnormalities in glucose and lipid metabolism, they carry an increased risk of heart disorders.[30]

Corticosteroids, used to reduce inflammation, can inhibit absorption of phosphorus and calcium, resulting in bone loss.[31] Since corticosteroids are filtered in the liver, long-time use can cause severe liver damage. These drugs have also been linked to *Candida albicans* infections.[32]

In addition to their possible dangerous effects, many drugs on the market today contain hidden cornstarch and lactose (a sugar found in milk). Although foods containing cornstarch and lactose must be labeled as such, no such law applies to drugs. In fact, the law in this case protects the drug companies. Trade Secrets legislation allows lactose and cornstarch to be labeled as "inert substances," and their presence may be concealed even from your doctor or pharmacist.[33] Today, over 1,500 drugs contain hidden cornstarch or lactose.

Very few prescription and over-the-counter drugs are symptom free. Again, the best advice is to focus on the problem that makes it necessary to take the drug. Dealing with the cause of the problem, rather than trying to alleviate the symptoms is the best and healthiest advice.

OVERHEATED FATS

It has long been reported that the breakdown product of charcoal-broiled beef causes cancer. A substance, benzo(a)pyrene, is produced during the breakdown of fat that drips from the steaks onto the hot coals. Smoke containing the benzo(a)pyrene then collects on the surface of the meat. The formation of these carcinogenic free radicals is dependent on the very high temperature required for the breakdown of fat.

When fats are overheated, especially through frying, charcoal broiling, and deep-frying, they can become rancid. The natural process of oxidation in the body, which produces free radicals (atoms lacking at least one electron), is made faster, much faster, when rancid fats are ingested.[34] There are many different kinds of free radicals, among them peroxide, hydroxyl group, and superoxide; and all are poisonous. Enzymes such as peroxidase, catalase, and superoxide dismutase are required to turn harmful free radicals back into useful products. As stated, enzymes depend on minerals to function optimally; when the body's mineral balance is upset by sugar, enzymes are unable to function correctly, and free radicals may be allowed to build up unimpeded.

If rancid fats are continually consumed, the enzymes necessary for preventing free-radical damage may become exhausted altogether. The body will be unable to deal with the free radicals normally, and the immune system must come to the rescue. It is best, therefore, not to overheat fats or to eat deep-fried food, particularly if the body chemistry is already unbalanced by sugar and other harmful substances.

OVERCOOKED FOODS

Many reports have indicated that eating red meat may give rise to certain forms of cancer of the digestive tract. However, a detailed study conducted at the University of California at Berkeley concludes that it is not the meat that causes damage, but rather the way in which it is cooked. The results of the study indicate that meat cooked at high temperatures (as when charcoal broiled, fried, or deep-fried) contains carcinogens. The best way to cook meat is slowly at low temperatures. Stews and pot roasts are recommended.[35]

All protein, whether wheat protein or vegetable protein (meats, vegetables, and legumes all have protein), has the same chemical configuration. Over the evolution of millions of years, our bodies have developed enzymes that match the protein molecules in our intestines. However, protein has a heat labile point—a temperature at which the protein becomes denatured and changes its configuration. Our enzymes are not designed to digest protein in this new configuration. As a result, noxious free radicals are produced. These free radicals cross the intestinal membranes, enter the bloodstream, and then must be fought by the immune system.[36]

Researchers Barbara Schneeman and George Dunaif, of the University of California at Davis, concluded that, no matter how delicious they may look, bread, milk, meat, eggs, and any other foods that are cooked to a golden brown have less nutritional value than their lightly cooked counterparts. Not only do overcooked foods have less food value, their nutrients are less digestible, and, therefore, less available.

Dr. Frances Pottenger had been researching cat diseases when, quite by accident, he discovered that the cats were affected by different diets. Local restaurants had been supplying him with cooked meat scraps to feed the cats, but after a while, they were not able to supply him with enough. Pottenger then obtained additional meat scraps—raw, not cooked—from a wholesaler. Soon, he was sur-

prised by the apparent good health of the cats who ate
the raw meat in contrast with those who ate the cooked
meat. The cats on the raw-food diet had thick and shiny
fur, produced healthy litters, and died of old age. The
cats who had eaten cooked food showed skeletal changes
and were unable to reproduce efficiently. They also
showed signs of respiratory problems, food allergies, and
dental disturbances. Pottenger found that the cats could be
so reduced in vitality by just one year of a diet considered
"adequate" for human consumption that they needed two
or three years to recover—if they recovered at all.[37] (Additional information on Dr. Pottenger's work with cats is
found beginning on page 106.)

The same effect has been noted in laboratory rats.
In one study, three groups of rats were fed prepared
nonfat dry milk as their only source of protein for four
weeks. One group was given the milk unheated. Another group was fed milk that had been heated to a
light brown. And the third group drank milk that had
been heated for forty-five minutes and was cocoa
brown. The rats on the unheated milk thrived, grew,
and gained weight. Those who ingested the light
brown milk took in less food and lost weight. The rats
who consumed the cocoa brown milk lost even more
weight. The researchers discovered that the browned
proteins stayed in the stomach longer than the lighter
proteins, indicating poor digestibility and poor absorption. As food gets overcooked, its chemical configuration changes and our enzymes are not able to
properly digest it.

The more raw foods you consume, the healthier the
diet. Raw foods contain more of the vitamins, minerals,
and enzymes so necessary for digestion and assimilation.

FOOD ADDITIVES

Food additives comprise another area with which the body's adaptive mechanism must deal. It is estimated that the average individual ingests at least one gallon of synthetic chemicals and additives, coloring agents, pesticides, and preservatives in a year's time. Artificial additives are used for one or more of the following purposes:

1. *To maintain or improve nutritional value,* such as through the addition of vitamins and minerals.

2. *To maintain freshness,* improving shelf life.

3. *To make food more appealing to sight* through the addition of stabilizers or artificial colors, *and to taste* through the addition of artificial flavors, sweeteners, MSG (monosodium glutamate), or other additives.

4. *To help in the processing or preparation of food* by acting as emulsifiers, stabilizers and thickeners, pH control agents, leavening agents, maturing and bleaching agents, anticaking agents, or humectants.[38]

Some addititives are safe, and some might even be beneficial; however, a number of people may experience negative reactions to them. Most symptoms of food-additive intolerance occur in the respiratory tract and skin. Common symptoms include respiratory infections, skin irritations, headaches, hyperkinesis, bladder urgency, joint and muscle pain, and diarrhea and other irritable bowel problems. Additives such as tartrazine and sulfites have been noted as frequent offenders,[39] as well as flavor enhancers such as monosodium glutamate.[40] Dr. Lewis Mayron tested chemicals used as coloring agents for foods and found that they destroyed both red blood cells and antibodies.[41]

The 1970s gave rise to a great deal of controversy over nitrates—the chemicals used to cure processed meats. Research showed that nitrosamines, the product of nitrites and nitrates, when combined with the stomach's naturally produced hydrochloric acid, are potent animal carcinogens. It is feared, therefore, that nitrates are likely to cause cancer in humans as well. (Although some vegetables are high in nitrites, they also contain ascorbic acid, which acts as an inhibitor of nitrosamine formation.)[42]

The federal government has attempted to lessen public exposure to nitrites, nitrates, and nitrosamines. Nitrate levels used in processed meats have been reduced, and, with a few exceptions, nitrate use in cured meats has been banned altogether. Nitrates in ham and bacon have been significantly reduced as well.

Here are a few steps you can take to further reduce your exposure to dangerous nitrosamines:

❑ *Take vitamin C.* Since ascorbic acid is a proven inhibitor of the formation of nitrosamines, taking vitamin C whenever nitrites are consumed will help. Vitamin supplements, cabbage, peppers, lettuce, and potatoes are all good providers of vitamin C.

❑ *Take vitamin E.* Research has indicated that naturally occurring vitamin E, found in cereals, grains, and vegetable fats, may also prevent the formation of nitrosamines.

❑ *Do not eat meats that have been cured with nitrites and nitrates.* Health food stores offer bacon, bologna, salami, hot dogs, and even hams that are chemical-free.

Your body is not meant to digest and metabolize chemicals easily. In particular, your liver must work hard to assimilate chemicals. It seems prudent not to tax your body any more than necessary. Allow me to share with you the following bit of advice: Before eating food, check its ingredient label. If you come across an ingredient that you cannot pronounce or spell (due to its obvious chemical origin), it would be wise not to put that food in your mouth.

ARTIFICIAL SWEETENERS

In an attempt to avoid sugar, many people have turned to nonsugar artificial sweeteners as substitutes. Aspartame and saccharin are the two types most commonly used. These artificial sweeteners, however, can be equally as harmful as sugar.

Asparatame

Originally sold under the brand names NutraSweet and Equal, aspartame is about 200 times sweeter than sugar. Aspartame is used in a number of diet sodas and soft drinks; it also comes a small packets and is stirred into coffee and tea, and sprinkled on bowls of cereal.

Aspartame is made up of three different substances: phenylalanine, aspartic acid, and methanol (wood alcohol). When digested, these substances are released into the bloodstream. It has been demonstrated that the effects of phenylalanine and tyrosine (both amino acids) are increased by aspartame in humans. High levels of these amino acids in the brain can negatively affect the synthesis of neurotransmitters and bodily functions that are controlled by the autonomic nervous system (e.g. blood pressure). Aspartame also inhibits the release of glucose into the bloodstream and induces the release of serotonin (an inhibitory transmitter) within the brain. High serotonin levels may affect behaviors such as sleep and hunger. Therefore, dieters may be only adding to their problems by drinking sodas with aspartame. Studies have also indicated that aspartic acid, when absorbed in excess, may cause endocrine disorders in mammals.

Methanol, a poisonous substance, is added during the manufacturing of aspartame. When aspartame-sweetened drinks are taken in hot weather or after an exercise session to replace body fluid, the intake of methanol can exceed 250 milligrams. That's thirty-two times higher than what the Environmental Protection Agency considers a safe consumption limit. The average aspartame content in a liter of cola drink is approximately 555 milligrams; of this amount, 56 milligrams are methanol.

Much medical research concludes that aspartame is not harmful to most people, and yet, the FDA has had numerous reports of seizures and other problems that have been linked to aspartame ingestion.[43] Dr. Richard Wurtman, professor of neuro-endocrine regulation at the Massachusetts Institute of Technology, Woodrow C. Monte, director of the Food Science and Nutrition Laboratory at Arizona State University, and the FDA have received thousands of complaints regarding aspartame consumption. In a report presented to the Senate Labor and Human Resources Committee, Dr. Wurtman reported the most common side effects linked to aspartame include dizziness, visual impairment, disorientation, ear buzzing, a high level of SGOT (an enzyme that breaks down protein into amino acids) in the blood, tunnel vision, loss of equilibrium, severe muscle aches, numbness of extremities, inflammation of the pancreas, episodes of high blood pressure, and eye hemorrhages.[44]

Individual cases of aspartame-related side effects regularly appear in medical journals. Written by medical doctors, these articles tell of problems such as hives, memory loss, attention deficit disorder, and headaches that have been linked to aspartame.[45] Although I have yet to learn of a study that involves the testing of aspartame on the immune or endocrine systems, I have learned that individuals with mood disorders are particularly sensitive to this artificial sweetener and should avoid it.[46]

Be cautious. Each chemical you ingest must be filtered by your liver. Over time, such "workouts" eventually exhaust the immune and endocrine systems. Stay away from such chemicals, strive to keep your body in homeostasis as much as possible.

Saccharin

The subject of controversy for many years, saccharin is currently sold with a label warning that its use may cause cancer. A ban on saccharin has been proposed but is currently being withheld pending further evidence. This artificial sweetener is found in Sweet 'N Low, Sprinkle Twin, and Sugar Twin.[47]

With the choice between sugar, aspartame, and saccharin, the public would be better off if it simply had its "sweet tooth" extracted. As the White Queen said in *Alice in Wonderland*, "The rule is, jam tomorrow and jam yesterday—but never jam today."

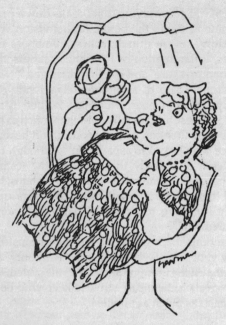

"Remember now, only my sweet tooth!"

MERCURY

Mercury poisoning from amalgam (silver) fillings have been implicated in conditions ranging from fatigue and nausea to headaches and double vision. One third of those with hypersensitivity to amalgam fillings run a subnormal body temperature, sometimes as low as 96°F. Mercury hypersensitivity can also be indicated by a metallic taste in the mouth and excessive saliva. Mercury poisoning can deplete the body's store of such minerals as lithium, which is used today to treat depression.

Interestingly enough, dentists appear to be particularly susceptible to mercury poisoning. Dr. DeWayne Ashmead, a biochemist and nutritionist, accidentally noticed high mercury levels in hundreds of dentists he had been testing for other minerals. Through urine samples, Dr. Ashmead found 10 percent of the dentists to be suffering from excessively high mercury levels.

Bringing the body back into balance can alleviate many of these symptoms. Removing the mercury toxicity from the mouth can help stop the unbalancing.

IN CONCLUSION

A variety of seemingly harmless substances and environmental stimuli can eventually become dangerous when the body chemistry is unbalanced by sugar or other abusive foods. Personally, once sugar had slowly but surely taken its toll on my immune system, many substances with which I had once lived in harmony became troublesome. Many things became intolerable.

As a child, I always enjoyed going on my parent's boat; but, as I grew older and began damaging the chemical balance of my body, I began to experience allergic symptoms from the dampness and mold. On windy days, the pollens in the air caused me to sneeze and made my eyes water. The dog I loved and had always been able to hug and pet, suddenly made my throat and ears itch whenever I went near him. When I filled my car with gas, the fumes caused me to feel fatigued. The perfume I had worn for years began to make me nauseous. Reading the newspaper made me fall asleep. I couldn't help but think the world was conspiring against me! In reality, it was my own dietary choices and abusive lifestyle that had created a condition that allowed environmental substances to upset my body chemistry even more.

My unbalanced body chemistry and compromised immune system caused each of my new maladies. It was only by removing sugar and other harmful substances from my life that I was able to help my body return to homeostasis and normalcy. Many people today become universal reactors—apparent victims of the twentieth-century lifestyle. However, far from being victims, they are creators of their own destabilized bodies by their poor choices over a lifetime. The good news is that people can change their condition, just as I did.

Another critical factor in maintaining homeostasis is stress, which is discussed in the following chapter.

7
Stress

S *tress* is a trendy word today. It is a topic that makes for great conversation at cocktail parties, appears week after week in books on the bestseller list, and is commonly discussed on television and radio talk shows. Psychologists, psychoanalysts, psychotherapists, hypnotherapists, and acupressurists all offer advice to help us deal with the stress in our lives. Stress-management seminars abound, not only in California, where such activity has been popular for many years, but throughout the United States.

Although the word *stress* is commonly used, *distress* might be a better word. Stress as a demanding event in one's life is so subjective that it is difficult to accurately measure its effects on health. What one person may consider stressful another might find stimulating. How a person responds to life's events, not the events themselves, is what influences his or her susceptibility to disease. Adequate coping with a high-stress life may reflect a psychological hardness, which is actually protective. Failure to cope well with stress, on the other hand, can impair a person's ability to fight off illness.[1]

The concept that psychological distress may predispose a person to physical illness is centuries-old but has only recently attracted the attention of the medical community at large. Psychoneuroimmunology is a new interdisciplinary field that focuses on the elusive mind-body connection. Information in this field is accumulated from areas of psychology, immunology, endocrinology, and the neurosciences.

PSYCHOLOGICAL DISTRESS

Distress has been found to have virtually the same effect on the body as sugar. It creates an imbalance in the body's calcium-phosphorus ratio. And as we have seen, whenever minerals change their relationship to one another, the body goes out of homeostasis. Enzymes do not work effectively, food does not digest properly, and the immune system must go into action.

When I researched the effects of sugar on the body's calcium-phosphorus ratio, I also did research on stress. I drew blood from two volunteers to determine their normal calcium-phosphorus ratio. I then had them immerse one hand in ice water for one minute, which is very stressful to the body. One volunteer immediately experienced back pain, which she hadn't felt in years. Afterward, I took another blood sample to check the calcium-phosphorus ratio. One volunteer's calcium level had risen while the phosphorus level dropped. In the other subject the opposite occurred: the level of phosphorus rose while the calcium level dropped. Of course, in both cases the ratio changed, which indicates how instantly distress (physical distress in this case) can change the body chemistry.

Evidence indicates that certain personality traits may predispose people to certain illnesses by weakening their immune processes. One such study involved 2,000 men who worked at a Chicago electric company. Twenty years earlier, these subjects had been given a questionnaire that rated "depression" levels. Those who had scored high on the questionnaire were found to have an increased cancer incidence and a higher cancer death rate than the others in the study. A second study involved 500 elderly men and women who participated in a survey that measured their level of "suspiciousness." During the succeeding fifteen years, those with highly suspicious natures also had significantly higher bouts with illnesses and incidents of death than others of the same age.[2]

Other studies have shown that a part of one's immune system becomes depressed during periods of distress. In particular, events such as academic examinations and social isolation (loneliness) cause a significant decrease in the natural-killer cell activity of the immune system.[3]

Researchers at the Albert Einstein College of Medicine of Yeshiva University, New York City, compared crises in the lives of two groups of children. One group included children with common minor ailments, the other group was of children with cancer. In the years before they were diagnosed, the children with cancer had experienced twice as many crises as those in the other group. These emotional upsets included such traumas as parental separation or divorce, death in the family, and change of school. In a different study, the emotional histories of thirty-three children suffering from leukemia were examined. Researchers found that thirty-one had experienced a traumatic emotional loss or change within two years before the leukemia was diagnosed. Half of these traumas had occurred six months before diagnosis.

Dr. Lawrence LeShan, a New York City psychologist, studied 450 adult cancer patients. He found that an incredible 72 percent had been either frustrated, lonely, or had experienced a major emotional loss anywhere from six months to eight years before their cancer was diagnosed. By comparison, Dr. LeShan found that only 10 percent of a control group of cancer-free people had a similar emotional pattern.

In another study, Dr. Steven Schleifer, a psychiatrist at New York's Mount Sinai School of Medicine, and his colleagues discovered a significant decline in the white blood cell activity of a person during the two-month period after losing a spouse. These cells, which are critical in fighting infection, continued to be suppressed for one year.[4]

Dr. Margaret Linn and her colleagues at the Veterans Administration Medical Center in Miami, Florida, conducted a study of heavy smokers—about half of whom had cancer. The researchers found no significant difference in the number of stressful events that had occurred in the lives of those who had cancer and those who did not. All of the study subjects had experienced various stressors, such as marital problems, business conflicts, family deaths, and everyday garden-variety challenges. However, Dr. Linn did discover that those smokers with cancer had perceived these stressful events as being negative. They felt more guilt and frustration over these situations than those subjects who had not developed cancer.

SUGAR AND PSYCHOLOGICAL DISTRESS

Recently, my daughter was in the hospital for minor surgery. After her operation, the doctor put her on a liquid diet. I was in her room one night when a nurse brought her dinner: Jell-O, ice cream, grape juice with corn sweetener, and tea with two packets of sugar. I was told by the dietician that this liquid diet had been approved by a committee of doctors and was used in hospitals all over the Los Angeles area. I assumed that children with serious illnesses such as cancer are also given these sweet foods during their hospital stay. Between the stress caused by simply being in the hospital and the sugar-laden diet, their little bodies are doubly challenged.

Like sugar, distress changes the mineral relationships in the body and exhausts the endocrine glands. It is the endocrine system that takes the initial beating when the body is under stress. The adrenal glands secrete adrenaline, which triggers a rise in blood pressure and an increase in blood flow to the muscles and the brain. A continued stimulation of the adrenals can exhaust these glands. And since adrenaline also stimulates the liver to convert its glycogen (stored sugar) into glucose (blood sugar), the pancreas must work to secrete insulin to convert the glucose into energy in the cells.

Constant stimulation and increased metabolic rate help deplete the biochemicals that go into the production of hormones, the glands' chemical messengers. Certain individuals, due to genetic weakness or poor diet, may experience a hypoglycemic response. Excess insulin circulating in the bloodstream lowers the blood sugar, depriving the brain of its principal fuel. The pancreas, which is particularly vulnerable when overworked, can eventually lose some or all of its insulin-producing capability, and diabetes may result.

The correlation between stress, sugar, and the endocrine glands is clearly seen in a study conducted in the former Soviet Union by Dr. I.I. Brekhman. Dr. Brekhman created stress in 246 female white rats by hanging them for eighteen hours by the fold of skin on the back of their necks. This stress produced several marked biochemical changes. The sugar content of the rats' blood increased from 86 milligrams to 128 milligrams per milliliter. There was an increased discharge of hormones into the blood, as well as a reduction in the amount of glycogen (stored sugar) in the liver.

At the onset of the study, the rats in both the control group and the experimental group had a stress index of zero. After the rats were stressed, the index rose to seven. When these same rats were fed white sugar, the stress index increased to nine. Each stressor caused a rise in the index. If we relate these study results to humans, we see that an individual can overload on stress from various sources. He or she might be experiencing emotional distress, then eat a candy bar, drink a cup of coffee, and inhale a hazardous chemical. While one stressor at a time might be safely handled, a collective amount can be too much for the body to deal with effectively.[5]

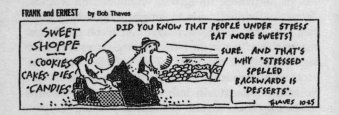

FRANK & ERNEST reprinted by permission of Newspaper Enterprise Association, Inc.

HANDLING DISTRESS

Obviously, it is important to limit the stressors in your life whenever possible. A divorce, loss of a job, high mortgage payments, trouble with in-laws—these are just a small sampling of common emotional challenges that are capable of causing physical illness. Just as stressful emotions can make us sick, positive emotions can help keep our bodies in balance and offset the damage of distress. There is much evidence that having positive emotions such as love and faith, enjoying a good sense of humor, and maintaining a positive mental attitude can help fight off illness.

The ways in which people bring joy to their lives varies from person to person, but I believe one thing to be a "given": we must feel and express love. Try to show love every day. Be open and honest with others about your feelings. Have fun. Try to laugh and enjoy life. This will help keep your body chemistry balanced and promote good health.

Distress certainly played an important role in the disease process in my body. From the time I was very young, I had to be the best at whatever I did. I had to be the one to collect the most newspapers in the school newspaper drive. It wasn't enough to be a United States Junior Tennis champion, I also had to be the fastest runner in my gym class. Becoming class president each year was an obsession. My drive to excel was relentless.

This need to excel, to be the best, was just a substitute for my self-esteem. I needed those outside achievements to feel good about myself. With the help of psychoanalysis, I finally learned to love and accept myself when I was in my thirties. I realized that I didn't have to win a tennis tournament in order to have friends. I didn't have to excel at anything. People were my friends just because they liked me.

The first change I noticed because of my new attitude was the way I played tennis. I didn't play any better, but suddenly it became so much easier and more enjoyable. My body just seemed to flow. It felt so good. No longer was someone looking over my shoulder asking, "What's the score?" Of course, no one had been doing that before, either. It was a pressure I had imposed on myself.

In the next chapter, we will take a look at the harmful effects of sugar on children.

8

Sugar, Spice, and Everything Nice

According to the age-old nursery rhyme, little girls are made of "sugar and spice and everything nice." Unfortunately, too many little girls (and little boys, too) *are* made of sugar—the sugar they eat. Do you know the average teenage boy eats twice as much sugar as people in any other age group? This means he eats an average of more than a cup of sugar a day.[1]

From the time we come into this world to the time we leave, sweeteners are present in most of the foods we eat. In the United States, the first nonmilk food a baby is likely to receive in the hospital is a 5-percent glucose-and-water solution.[2] Some baby milk formulas include sugar. Children are often rewarded with sugary treats: "Eat your dinner and you will get dessert." Some behavior-modification classes reward children with candy when they have finished an assignment or displayed good behavior. How many pediatricians reward their patients with lollipops? To raise money for local sports teams and organizations, children commonly sell sweet treats such as Girl Scout cookies and chocolate bars. And aren't bake sales at schools and churches traditional fundraising events? The list goes on.

THE LINK BETWEEN SUGAR
AND CHILDREN'S HEALTH

A variety of health problems in children have been implicated by sugar. Such problems include hyperactivity, obesity, and, of course, allergies.

Dr. William Crook, pediatrician and author of *The Yeast Connection*, feels that he has an understanding of the role that sugar plays in the hyperactivity of children. Through research, he found that gastrointestinal growth and invasion of *Candida albicans* was approximately 200 times greater in mice who received dextrose in their feedings, than in a control group of mice who received no dextrose. When a person has an overgrowth of candida in the intestines there is more gut permeability. This means that when candida is present in the gut, undigested or partially digested food can get from the intestines into the bloodstream. Along with a number of other problems, this undigested food can cause hyperactivity.[3]

The information on the link between sugar and hyperactivity in children is controversial. Some research suggests sugar causes hyperactivity and aggressiveness in children, while other research indicates that there is no connection.[4]

Forty-eight children and their families were involved in a recent study conducted by medical investigators at Vanderbilt University in Nashville, Tennessee. During the nine-week study, the children were given food that had been prepared both with and without sugar or aspartame. The researchers carefully observed the children, noting any differences in their general behavior and mental capabilities after they had eaten both the sweetened and unsweetened meals. Their evaluations indicated no evidence that sugar had any adverse effect on the children's behavior.

However, it is important to note that the sugar ingested was in small amounts and given over the period of an entire day. In other words, none of the children binged on the sugar. Also, the total amount of sugar ingested on any given day fell within the range of normal; unusually large amounts were not eaten. And the diet itself was nutritionally sound; it did not include food colorings, preservatives, or other additives.[5] It was not at all representative of the typical American diet.

Other studies have indicated that sugar certainly does cause hyperactivity in children. In one double-blind crossover study, a dose of sugar equivalent to that found in an average 12-ounce can of soda pop (approximately ten teaspoons) was shown to disrupt the performance of preschool children. Behavioral differences were most pronounced forty-five to sixty minutes after ingestion. During structured testing situations, the children displayed decreased performance. They also showed increased inappropriate behavior during free-play situations.[6]

The research of Dr. Alex Schauss indicates that when sugar is removed from a child's diet, school grades go up. In addition to sugar, when sucrose and food additives were removed from children's diets there were significant gains in scholastic national rankings based on the California Achievement Tests. The four-year period that showed scholastic gains were the same four years in which the schools made major dietary revisions in their school lunch

CLOSE TO HOME By John McPherson

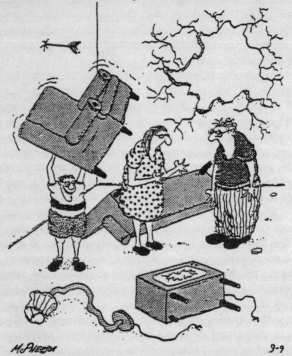

"He does not have a discipline problem! He's just had a little too much sugar, that's all."

programs. Foods that contained sucrose or additives were no longer served. Before the dietary changes, the 803 schools involved averaged 41 percentile in the scholastic national ranking; after four years, the mean academic performance rose to 51 percentile. New York City schools that had undergone the same dietary changes in their school lunch programs saw their scholastic average move from 11 percent below the national average to 5 percent above the national mean.[7]

Obesity in children is a another growing problem worldwide. Significant factors influencing weight gain include increased TV watching, poor dietary habits—fast foods, sugar intake, processed foods—and poor physical education programs at school. Only 36 percent of our children are involved in a daily athletic program at school. Children must learn proper lifestyle habits in the home to reduce the risk of health problems such as obesity.[8] Unfortunately, all too often, it is the overweight moms and dads who have encouraged their children's poor eating habits, lack of exercise, and passive recreational choices.

If you have an obese or overweight child, begin by removing the sugar, wheat, and dairy products from his or her diet.[9] Encourage your child to exercise regularly. Along with a health-care professional, create a daily exercise program to meet the specific needs of your child. Restrict the time spent on "nonactive activities," such as watching television, playing video games, and working on a computer. You will be amazed at the physical as well as psychological differences that will follow.

WHAT YOU CAN DO

So where do I stand? It is simple, so simple. If your child has a hard time falling asleep or staying asleep, cannot concentrate in school or at home, has low grades in school, suffers with allergies, is prone to headaches, is hyperactive or listless, is overweight, cannot go for more than four hours without eating, has a hard time keeping friendships, or has colds or bacterial infections more than once a year, I suggest that you remove sugar (all forms) from his or her diet for two weeks. In this short time, I think you will see a positive change in your child. Place the child on Food Plan III, found on page 163.

Early childhood symptoms can mean degenerative diseases as an adult. Following Food Plan III may help alleviate some of your child's symptoms and put him or her on the road to good health. There is nothing your child can lose besides poor eating habits. And as an added bonus, think of the money you'll save by cutting ice cream, cakes, and candies from your grocery list.

I have known many children who have had one or more of the above-mentioned symptoms. Once sugar had been removed from their diets, seemingly miraculous changes suddenly occurred—physical symptoms diminished or disappeared, energy levels increased, concentration levels became stronger, and self-esteem improved.

Notice that Food Plan III eliminates milk and wheat products from the diet. Many people are allergic to these products because they have continually eaten them with too much sugar. For example, wheat is made into donuts, cakes, pies, and cookies. Milk is made into products such as ice cream, cheesecakes, and puddings. Many people have become allergic to wheat and milk due to the continual eating of these sugary products. We can make ourselves allergic to any food we continually eat with sugar.

If your child has been on Food Plan III for two weeks and is still displaying negative physical or psychological symptoms, don't take him or her off the food plan. You must determine more specifically the cause(s) of the allergic reactions. The Body Chemistry Test Kit (see page 161) can help you figure out the cause of your child's allergies. Once the "culprit foods" are identified, remove them from your child's diet. (Of course, always eliminate sugar.) At this point, your child should begin to display positive results.

I love working with children because, unlike many adults, they have not abused their bodies for an extended period of time. Their bodies also respond quickly. For example, when an allergic substance is removed from a child's body, he or she will quickly return to homeostasis. It takes just a few days to see a difference. And don't forget about your child's psychological health. Like adults, children have psychological needs that require attention. All four arenas of life (see page 155) must be addressed.

Remember one thing, loving your children is more important than nagging them not to eat sugar. Children can change their diets as young adults and regain much physical health; but if they have not received proper love, they will have difficulty gaining a healthy psychological outlook. My children were around age seven and eleven when I realized the negative effects sugar was having on my health and the health of my family. In response, I simply removed sugar from our home, all of it. I knew my children occasionally ate sugar when they went out, but I didn't rant and rave when they did. Actually I said very little. I let my actions do the talking for me instead. My children watched as I got rid of the sugar and sugar-sweetened products from our household. Best of all, they witnessed a dramatic transformation in me as my chronic allergy symptoms disappeared and there was a noticeable improvement in the way I felt and acted. Seeing these positive changes in my health made a lasting impression on my children, who became aware, firsthand, of the harmful effects of sugar.

You have seen how many ways there are to upset the body's chemical balance—both physical and psychological. The next chapter offers a number of plans to help you change your abusive lifestyle and regain and/or maintain good health.

9

A Practical Plan for Attaining and Maintaining Good Health

It is paradoxical that in a time of technological advances, material abundance, and extended life spans, growing numbers of Americans are experiencing more and varied forms of health breakdowns. One out of every two persons today develops cardiovascular disease; one out of three, cancer; one out of five, diagnosable mental illness; and one out of five, diabetes. Birth defects are on the rise, and recent studies reveal that our children aren't as strong physically as children were fifty years ago. Scholastic test scores continue to fall. New and unprecedented forms of disease are occurring. Allergies and low-energy conditions abound. The cost for health care (which is really "disease care") is now a staggering three billion dollars a day.

Clearly, the quality of health is decreasing, and an increasing number of people are not responding well, or in a lasting way, to appropriate medical care. Our ancestors, who led less materialistic, less stressful lifestyles, had stronger bodies by contast. It is, however, possible for people today to escape the perils of the modern lifestyle, as well as avoid the downward spiral of degenerative disease. This chapter is devoted to showing you how, based upon the principles we have discussed.

In the preceding chapters you have seen how sugar as well as a variety of other substances and stress can disturb your body chemistry and lead to degenerative disease. The good news is that the damage can be reversed. Once you have licked the sugar habit and have started following the guidelines and plans presented in this chapter, you will be able to build up your body's enzymes, your endocrine and immune systems, and, in fact, your health in general.

Understand the following principles, which form a solid foundation for maintaining good health:

- Both disease and good health are the result of the condition of the body's chemistry. Health breakdowns result from an unbalanced body chemistry—a body whose minerals are out of their proper relationships.

- Your body chemistry may become unbalanced quickly. Depending on your adaptive abilities, your chemistry may stay unbalanced or rebalance just as quickly.

- The extent of any health breakdown is determined by the degree and duration of the chemical imbalance.

- The only difference between a well person and a person with a health breakdown is that the well person can efficiently rebalance his or her body chemistry.

■ After a health breakdown, the way in which your body responds to appropriate medical care depends on the ability of your body chemistry to rebalance.

■ Through conscious and unconscious choices, you can control your body's chemical balance.

Understanding and acting upon these principles will help you to regain and/or maintain good health.

THE FOUR ARENAS

There are four "arenas" in which we act that produce basic effects on our chemical balance. Let's take a closer look at each arena as illustrated in Figure 9.1. Through them, we can learn the steps necessary to improve our lifestyles.

Arena I: Our Interpretations

Arena I involves the choices we make in interpreting what we and others do, think, and say. Our minds can get in the way of good health. Our emotions, the way we feel—good or bad—can change our mineral relationships and alter our chemical balance.

It is important to observe the language we use and pay attention to the ways we upset our body chemistry through what we say, how we think, and how we act. To illustrate this concept, I want you to close your eyes and picture a lemon—a plump, fresh, bright yellow, freshly cut lemon. Now bring the lemon to your nose and smell it. Next lick it. Finally, slowly take a big juicy bite out of

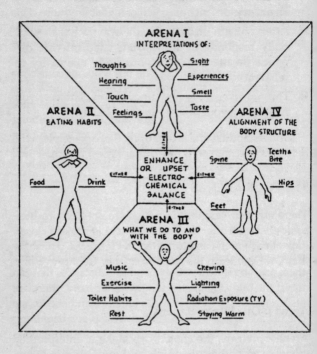

Figure 9.1. The Four Arenas: Electrochemical Balance.

it. I'll bet you are salivating by now! Can you see how
simply thinking of that lemon altered your body chemistry? In the same way, an angry or depressing thought,
or a negative emotion can affect your chemical balance,
throwing your body out of homeostasis.

Once a decision is made to change a harmful lifestyle, you must commit to that action. Telling a loved
one or a friend about the action is helpful. Let's say

you want to become more patient; toward this end, you make a commitment not to yell or swear anymore. This goal will be easier to achieve if you share your commitment with someone else. This gives you a greater sense of obligation.

As individuals, we must find out why our conscious and subconscious sometimes works against us. When we upset our body chemistry, the physical imbalance can affect our minds and prevent us from thinking clearly and rationally. Little problems can become big problems. Things that normally do not upset us can bring on feelings of anger or rage. When the body is upset, the mind can become upset as well.

Arena II: Eating Habits

Arena II deals with what we choose to ingest—foods, beverages, and drugs. As discussed in earlier chapters, there are foods and a variety of other substances that can upset the body chemistry. On the other hand, there are also a number of foods that can enhance and encourage chemical balance. Three detailed food plans beginning on page 162 are designed to help you choose those foods that are best for you.

As a former sugarholic and chocoholic, I can still remember the pleasure (misdirected, as I know now) I would get from eating sugar. I'm not sure how, when, or why it happened, but the thought process that once directed me toward sweets has changed. Now I think in terms of eating foods that don't upset my body chemistry. I enjoy food just as much as I used to, and possibly more. I certainly can eat more, because I've given up all those refined foods with so little bulk and so many calories. You can do the same.

Arena III: What We Do To and With Our Bodies

Arena III deals with body mechanics, which include such things as proper exercise, good toilet habits, and even how we chew our food. Through good habits, you can help bring an unbalanced body back into alignment.

Follow the guidelines presented below:

■ Chew each bite of food at least twenty times. Digestion begins in the mouth; an enzyme in saliva starts the process. Help your digestive system by chewing your food well.

■ When nature calls—answer. Your body is telling you it wants to get rid of waste. If you ignore the urge to go to the bathroom, for even a half hour, the urge may pass. Undigested food that stays in the colon too long can become toxic. The immune system must then deal with the by-products of putrefaction.

■ Drink enough water to stay hydrated. Be sure to drink between meals.

■ Regularly, do some form of exercise that uses opposite arm-leg movements. This includes running, swimming, walking, or any exercise in which your arms swing back and forth in a balancing motion. Aerobic exercise is great. If you don't do aerobics, then deep-breathe to get air as far into the lungs as possible. Always begin your exercise regimen by stretching.

■ Almost everything connected to an electrical circuit radiates an electromagnetic field while it operates. These fields create low-frequency radiation, which can negatively influence health depending on the strength and duration of the exposure.[1] It is, therefore, prudent to keep a safe distance from sources of such radiation. For example:

- Don't sleep within three feet of an electrical clock.
- While watching television, sit at least ten feet from the set.
- While working on a computer, maintain a distance of at least three feet from the monitor.
- Keep a distance of at least six feet from a microwave that is on.
- Do not use electric blankets.

■ Tungsten-halogen light bulbs and most fluorescent light sources emit harmful ultraviolet rays. Sitting under or near such light sources can result in harmful effects on the body. Use full-spectrum light bulbs, instead. Full-spectrum lighting is the most natural type.[2]

■ Studies show that listening to loud hard-rock music can negatively change the body chemistry in some people. If this or other music has such an effect on you—if it makes you anxious or nervous—by all means, stop listening to it.

■ Assure yourself six to eight hours of quiet sleep per night, and sleep warm. (Being too hot or too cold can upset the body chemistry.)

These simple suggestions should help you to lighten the negative load you may be carrying as the result of a modern-day lifestyle.

Arena IV: Alignment of Body Structure

When any part of the body is out of alignment—jaws, neck, spine, hips, or feet—you will experience distress.

Distress, in turn, upsets mineral relationships. A chiro-
proctor can realign your body. If the other arenas of your
body are in balance, the realignment will likely hold.
However, if you are not functioning well in other arenas,
if mineral relationships are already upset, tissue integrity will be compromised. Although a chiropractor may
make an adjustment, it may not hold. The four arenas
are interrelated; each must be balanced before health
can be achieved.

EXTENDED APPLICATION
OF THE FOUR ARENAS

This book is not intended as a handbook or manual in
response to all ailments. It should, however, be useful to
most people most of the time. Its concepts provide the
basis for a response to any disease, no matter how
serious. Certainly no one will ever be harmed by removing sugar, fat, and processed and other abusive foods
from his or her diet. The extent to which the concepts in
this book must be applied depends on one's genetic
blueprint, the length of time and severity of the abuse,
and the nature of the resulting condition.

Recent research on AIDS shows that an approach
similar to the one outlined in this book has been used
to improve the immune system and the general condition of AIDS patients. Patients use a variety of
methods that dealt with all four arenas. Arena I activities include involvement in ongoing support
groups and psychotherapy sessions, maintenance of
a personal journal, practice of relaxation techniques—meditation, biofeedback, self-hypnosis,
visualization—and the investigation of philosophy
and religion. Arena II activity includes following one

of the food plans from this chapter (minus any reactive foods), supplemented by vitamins, minerals, and herbal preparations. Arenas III and IV include activities such as taking saunas to cleanse and detoxify, having massages (including rolfing—deep muscle and organ massage), and doing aerobic exercise. Taking homeopathic remedies and colonics, and having chiropractic adjustments are also part of this regimen.

We are all unique individuals; and each of us responds differently to different therapies. For some people, simple modifications in lifestyle can greatly improve their health. Other people need to explore many different modalities to help their bodies heal.

TESTING FOR HOMEOSTASIS

It is possible for you to discover those arenas that are giving you trouble, which foods are most likely to create imbalance in your body chemistry, and how well you are maintaining your health. Through use of the Body Chemistry Test Kit, you can discover if the foods you eat are being digested and metabolized properly. If you are experiencing stress, this kit will help you determine if that stress has become distress and is upsetting your body chemistry.

The test works by measuring the amount of calcium in the urine. It lets you know if you are secreting too much, too little, or a normal amount of calcium. Since calcium works only in relation to phosphorus, this test also indicates whether the phosphorus level is too high for the calcium present (no calcium will show up in the urine), whether the phosphorus level is too low for the calcium present (too much calcium will show up in the urine), or if there is a correct amount of calcium for the phosphorus present (there will be a normal amount of calcium in the urine).

Although the test detects only calcium, if the calcium-phosphorus ratio is out of balance, the rest of the minerals in the body are also out of balance. When the calcium-phosphorus ratio is properly balanced, the rest of the body's minerals are balanced also. When minerals are in the right relationship, they function optimally, as do the vitamins and enzymes.

This home test kit for monitoring your body's chemical balance comes with a booklet that explains its use. (See page 243 for ordering information.)

THE FOOD PLANS

The following food plans are effective in helping your body achieve homeostasis. If you experience symptoms such as headaches, allergies, joint pains, general fatigue (especially after meals), or high blood pressure, or if you have a degenerative disease, you might start out by following Food Plan I. If, after a week, your symptoms are still present, or you are unable to maintain homeostasis (as determined by the Body Chemistry Test), try Food Plan II, which is more restrictive. Again, if symptoms still persist, go on to Food Plan III.

Also, be aware that by following the food plans, you may initiate withdrawal symptoms from the addictive foods, which are no longer in your diet. Omitting these foods can result in such painful symptoms as fever, depression, headaches, chills, anger, and fatigue. In some people, symptoms may last two or three days; for others, the symptoms may last a week.

Food Plan I

1. Avoid all foods in Categories IV and V (see food lists starting on page 165). Eat any other food.

2. If you are not beginning to feel better after being on Food Plan I for seven days, your body chemistry may require a more comprehensive food plan. Therefore, proceed with Food Plan II.

Food Plan II

1. Avoid all foods in Categories III, IV, and V (see food lists starting on page 165). For meals, eat foods found in Category I. Foods in Category II may be eaten in small amounts and only between meals.

2. If you are still not experiencing better health after being on Food Plan II for seven days, you may need an even more restrictive food plan. Proceed with Food Plan III.

Food Plan III

It is clear that your unbalanced body chemistry involves more than just the foods common to body chemistry upset. Food Plan III is designed to provide complete nutrients to your body in their most bio-available form. Foods in this plan are the ones most people can digest, metabolize, and assimilate easily. The procedures and foods of Food Plan III are the least stressful to your body chemistry. Do the following:

1. For fourteen days, eat only those foods from Category I (see food lists starting on page 165). Eat one small portion from each food group four or five

times a day. Remember to follow the Health-Promoting Eating Habits beginning on page 171.

2. If, after fourteen days you are still not experiencing relief of symptoms and have addressed all four arenas, you'll need to see a qualified practitioner who can test your blood for food sensitivities. You must find foods that do not upset your body chemistry.

FOOD CATEGORIES

The following food categories should be followed according to Food Plans I, II, and III (pages 163–164.)

Category I

When properly prepared and eaten, the following foods are best tolerated by those with an unbalanced body chemistry.

GREEN LEAFY VEGETABLES	GREEN VEGETABLES	ROOT VEGETABLES
Artichoke	Alfalfa	Jicama
Brussels sprouts	Asparagus	Onion
Cabbage	Avocado	Parsnip
Kale	Broccoli	Potato
Lettuce (all)	Celery	Radish
Spinach	Chinese pea pods	Rutabaga
	Okra	Turnip

YELLOW/WHITE VEGETABLES	HERBS / CONDIMENTS	
Cauliflower	Arrowroot	Lime
Corn	Basil	Mustard
Cucumber	Bay leaf	Nutmeg
Squash (all)	Black pepper	Olive oil
	Butter	Oregano
	Caraway	Parsley
ORANGE/PURPLE/ RED VEGETABLES	Chili pepper	Rose hips
Beet	Chive	Rosemary
Carrot	Cilantro	Safflower oil
Eggplant	Dill	Sage
Pumpkin	Garlic	Sesame oil
Sweet potato	Ginger	Sunflower oil
Tomato	Horseradish	Tarragon
	Lemon	Thyme

*Although avocado is a fruit, it is included in Category I foods.

Category I (continued)

FISH		BEANS/GRAINS
Anchovy	Red snapper	Azuki beans
Bass	Salmon	Barley
Catfish	Sardine	Bean sprouts
Clam	Scallop	Black beans
Cod	Shark	Black-eyed peas
Crab	Shrimp	Buckwheat
Flounder	Sole	Garbanzo beans
Haddock	Swordfish	Green beans
Halibut	Trout	Green peas
Mackerel	Tuna	Kidney beans
Oyster	Any other fish	Lentils
Perch		Lima beans
		Millet
MEATS / POULTRY*		Navy beans
Bacon		Oats
Beef		Pinto beans
Chicken		Red beans
Chicken eggs		Rice, brown
Duck		(preferred)
Lamb		Rice, white
Liver, beef and chicken		Rice, wild
Pheasant		Rye
Pork		Soybeans
Turkey		Split peas
Venison		White beans

* Hopefully, you will be able to eat meat and poultry from free-range, organically fed animals.

If you are a vegetarian, eliminate foods from the Fish and the Meat/Poultry categories. Combine the beans and grains for complete protein.

Category II

Some body chemistries are sensitive to these otherwise wholesome foods.

FRUITS
Apples
Apricots
Bananas
Cantaloupe
Coconuts
Cranberries
Dates
Figs
Grapes
Guava
Melons (all)
Nectarines
Papayas
Peaches
Pears
Pineapples
Raspberries
Strawberries
Watermelon

NUTS/SEEDS	
Almonds	Pecans
Brazil nuts	Pistachios
Chestnuts	Poppy seeds
Hazelnuts	Safflower seeds
Hickory nuts	Sunflower seeds
Macadamia nuts	Walnuts

HERBS/CONDIMENTS	
Anise seeds	Cream of tartar
Chicory	Paprika
Clove	Spearmint

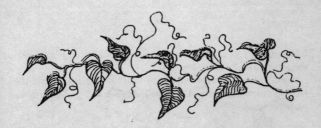

Category III

Overcooking, overeating, and eating foods with sugar have turned these normally well-tolerated foods into potentially abusive ones for some people. This includes those who have already compromised their systems through continued abuse.

GRAINS	DAIRY	
Wheat bran	Buttermilk	Milk, cow's
Wheat germ	Cheese (all)	Whey
White flour	Cream cheese	Yogurt
Whole wheat		

FUNGI	MISCELLANEOUS	
Mushrooms	Carob	Honey
Yeast, baker's	Cinnamon	Hops
Yeast, brewer's	Coffee, regular	Molasses
	Coffee, decaffein-	Peppermint
FRUITS	ated	Processed foods
Grapefruit	Cola bean	Rice syrup
Mango	Corn gluten	Salt
Orange	Cornstarch	Tea
Tangerine	Curry	Vanilla
	Fructose	

NUTS/SEEDS
Cashews
Peanuts

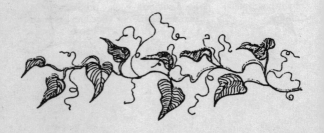

Category IV

The following items are always abusive to human body chemistry. Only those who remain adaptive can rebalance after frequent exposure to the items listed here. The more Category IV foods consumed, the more rapid the deterioration in the body chemistry.

Alcohol	Cocoa	Malt
Beet sugar	Corn sugar	Maple sugar
Cane sugar	Corn syrup	Saccharin

Category V

Items on the following list have been proven to unbalance the body chemistry. It serves your good health to either stay away from these items or to use them sparingly and with caution. Some are used as preservatives, fillers, or coloring agents in processed foods. Be sure to read labels!

Acetaminophen	Drugs: over-the-	Ibuprofen
Aspirin	counter, pre-	MSG (monosodium
Baking powder	scription, and	glutamate)
BHT (butylated	street	Petroleum by-
hydroxytoluene)	Food coloring	products
Caffeine	Formaldehyde	Sodium benzoate
		Tobacco

SIMPLE SUGGESTIONS
FOR BREAKFAST AND SNACKS

People who are on Food Plan III and eat only Category I foods sometimes have difficulty with ideas for breakfast. Here are a few suggestions, many of which are also great as snacks.

- In the evening, cook some potatoes then refrigerate them. In the morning, slice the potatoes and sauté in butter.
- Baked potato with butter, guacamole, or puréed beans.
- Corn tortilla with butter, tomatoes, scrambled egg, and/or guacamole.
- Oatmeal with butter.
- Cream of Rice with butter.
- Rice cakes with sliced avocado, tomato, onion, green pepper, or cucumber.
- One-egg omelet with sliced tomato and diced vegetables (potato, green pepper, and onion are good choices).
- One-egg ranchero with corn tortilla.
- Cooked rice with butter.
- Steamed sweet potato with butter. Sweet potatoes are also good cold. They taste like candy.
- One cup of popped corn.
- Leftover rice heated with grated carrots, frozen peas, frozen lima beans, and butter. (This is my personal favorite.)

HEALTH-PROMOTING EATING HABITS

Regardless of which food plan you are following, be sure to observe the following general health-promoting eating habits:

❑ Chew each mouthful of food at least twenty times.

❑ Do not wash foods down with liquids. Swallow your food before taking a drink.

❑ Consume portions you can easily digest.

❑ If you are emotionally upset or disturbed, eat smaller portions and chew your food longer than usual.

❑ Do not overcook your food.

❑ At each meal consume as much raw food as you do cooked.

❑ Rather than eating large meals less often, consume smaller meals more often.

❑ Examine each meal and snack from the following viewpoint: "Will any part of this meal upset my body chemistry?"

❑ Eating small portions from a number of foods is far better than eating one large serving of a particular food.

Following these good eating habits will lessen the incidents of body chemistry imbalance and facilitate more efficient digestion, assimilation, and utilization of nutrients. In addition, you will be supporting your body's ability to rebalance its chemistry in spite of other lifestyle insults. Finally, your response to appropriate medical care will be enhanced.

CONCLUSION

As you can see, what you *do not* put in your mouth is as important (or possibly more important) than what you *do*. You can sit down to a "perfect nutritious meal" that includes foods from Food Plan III, but if you finish that meal with a piece of cake, you will be canceling the meal's nutritional goodness. The sugar in the cake will upset the body's mineral balance, making the nutrients from the meal less available.

We all have cravings and addictions. However, ultimately, you are the one who is responsible for what goes into (and what does not go into) your mouth.

You are also responsible for what comes out of your mouth, as well as what you think and how you feel. Again, you might sit down to that "perfect nutritious meal," but if you are distressed, depressed, angry, or if you are harboring any other negative emotion, you will cancel the meal's nutritional goodness.

Health or disease. The choice is yours.

10
Self-Help
Techniques

B y now you should have a good idea of the negative effects of both sugar and stress on the body's homeostasis—effects that can lead to degenerative disease. I hope you have made a commitment to improving your diet and lifestyle, and that you follow the lifestyle guidelines and one of the food plans that are offered in Chapter 9. Nevertheless, if you have been a sugarholic, you may still find it difficult to lick the sugar habit entirely. The suggestions in this chapter will ease you through those cravings you are likely to experience during the withdrawal period.

So many times I have been asked why people crave sugar. New research might give the poor sufferer a reason. In the liver and certain tissues of the body, glucose is stored in the form of glycogen. When our blood glucose drops a little, our adrenal glands help by taking this stored sugar (glycogen), converting it back to glucose, and returning it to the bloodstream; this keeps our body from feeling the effects of low blood sugar (hypoglycemia). Sluggish adrenal glands, however, are slow to convert glycogen to glucose in time of need, and the craving for something sweet becomes overwhelming.

Insulin is secreted by the pancreas after we eat sugar to help remove the excess sugar from the bloodstream and store it in the cells. When the amount of necessary insulin has been secreted, it is the adrenal hormone's job to send a message to the pancreas to stop producing insulin. Sluggish adrenals will be late in this function, allowing production of too much insulin with a resultant excessive lowering of the blood sugar. Low blood sugar causes people to have strong sugar cravings, as well as headaches, fatigue, lightheadedness, perspiration, nausea, anger, and/or depression. It seems like a vicious cycle and it is. Distress, caffeine, and sugar all stress the pancreas, which, in turn, causes the adrenals to become overworked. Eventually, the result is sluggish or inadequate adrenal function. Elimination of these culprits is the key. The result will be a more stable blood sugar.

Sugar is as addictive as a drug. The taste for sweets can lead to a craving for more of the same, just the way a drug can create cravings. Drugs upset the body's homeostasis mechanism so completely that, in a struggle to get back to normal, the addict craves only another dose of the same drug. The more you have, the more you want, and the more manufacturers will provide.

WHAT YOU CAN DO

The following suggestions are provided to help you combat cravings and addictions.

Don't Keep Sugar-Laden Foods at Home

Throw away any foods that contain sugar; pitch them right out. Then, if you need a "fix," you will have to drive to the store to feed your habit. This will give you time to think and possibly change your mind. Or, buy only enough to satisfy your craving. Don't buy more than you can eat at the moment. Buy the smallest size of whatever it is you crave, and throw out what you don't eat. Better wasted outside the body than inside.

Remove Corn From Your Diet

Since so much of the sugar in processed foods comes from a corn base, I suggest you leave corn out of your diet until you have given up sugar for two months. If you have been eating a lot of sugar, you are probably allergic to corn.

Any form of corn—cornstarch, corn sweetener, corn bread, corn on the cob—can bring on a craving. In fact, any form of food to which you are allergic can cause a craving. Avoid such foods.

Battle Hypoglycemia With Carbohydrates

If you should go into a hypoglycemic state and experience symptoms such as fatigue, perspiration, dizziness, or lightheadedness, you may be tempted to eat sugar, thinking that it will bring your blood sugar level back to normal. Remember that this will help you only for the moment and will hurt you in the long run. An influx of sugar may lift the blood sugar level so high that it has to come crashing down again.

Instead of sugar, eat complex carbohydrates such as potatoes, whole wheat bread, crackers, or even nuts. After eating these foods, it may take longer for your blood sugar level to return to normal, but it will avoid the yo-yo effect that sugar produces.

Snack on Healthy Foods

Snacks don't have to be unhealthful. Steam a few white potatoes, sweet potatoes, yams, squash, and other foods containing complex carbohydrates. Keep these in your refrigerator along with raw foods such as green and red peppers, jicama, carrots, and celery. Then, during those snack attacks, you will have good healthy foods readily available to choose from.

Always Read Labels

If food labels contain words that you cannot pronounce (due to their obvious chemical origin) don't put that food in your mouth. Also, be on the lookout for any words on ingredient lists that mean sugar. This would include, for instance, honey, maple syrup, corn syrup, corn sweetener, dextrine, barley malt, rice syrup, glucose, sucrose, and dextrose.

As you probably know, ingredients must be listed on product labels according to their predominance; don't be fooled by a product that lists corn sweetener as the third ingredient, brown sugar as the fourth, and dextrose as the fifth. This is a deceptive method of dealing with a lot of sugar in a product. If these three types of sugar were combined on the product's ingredient list, sugar might very well be the first (most predominant) ingredient on the label.

Eat Protein in Small Portions

Protein is absorbed and simultaneously broken down into amino acids. This makes possible the release of glycogen (stored sugar), which raises the blood glucose level. If the blood sugar level is elevated, it must come down; and as the level falls, you may crave sweets.

Next time you get a sugar craving, think about what you ate at your last meal; if it included a large portion of meat or fish, you might try cutting down on the portion next time. The body needs protein, but eat small portions at each meal, rather than a large portion at one meal. Some forms of protein may trigger cravings while others may not. This is another good time to get in touch with your body and pay attention to the signals it is giving you.

Get Help From Your Friends

Try going on the buddy system with a friend who is cutting out sugar from his or her diet or just trying to lose weight. Phone your buddy when you are feeling in need of a little support. Besides, support from a friend always feels good, whether it is for help or just for pure friendship.

If you are craving sugar because of loneliness or depression, telephoning a friend should help your state of mind, too. And, if you are a person who needs to be scolded into refraining from your bad habit, then pick someone who will do that for you. On the other hand, you may simply need someone who is willing to listen to you. And if you are responsible for being someone else's buddy, you may be less apt to cheat yourself.

Exercise!

Exercising shuts down the appestat—the mechanism in the brain that controls appetite. Following vigorous exercise, most people are not hungry. So exercise helps a person stay fit, not only because it burns calories, but because it decreases one's appetite.

Avoid Artificial Sweeteners

In a number of laboratory tests, rats were given saccharin. Their bodies were fooled into thinking the sweetener was sugar, and they produced a boost of insulin. This is one reason why artificial sweeteners are poor aids for weight watchers and sugarholics; they are not good substitutes for sugar.

If you find yourself giving in to a candy craving, know that many health food stores carry candies sweetened with maltose, sorbitol, or other forms of complex natural sugars (sugars that need some digesting and breaking down into simple sugars). Choose these over products made with artificial sweeteners such as saccharin and NutraSweet, and certainly over those made with white ganulated sugar, which get into the bloodstream quickly—too quickly.

Substitute Carob for Chocolate

There are many carob candies on the market today and most are made without sugar. Be aware, however, that most contain hydrogenated fat, which is difficult for the body to utilize. Try making your own candy from powdered carob instead. And be sure to try the luscious Carob Mousse (page 197) and the Spicy Carob Brownies (page 199).

Avoid Temptation

There are certain situations in which you may be more likely to eat sugar, and you should avoid these situations whenever possible. This doesn't mean you should quit your job, but you might change the place where you eat lunch or take a walk when the fast-food truck comes.

Use Delaying Tactics

When you have a sugar craving, try to put off satisfying that urge for fifteen minutes, then a half hour, then an hour. Substitute the time with positive activities. Relaxation techniques work for some people, while others find strength in meditation and prayer. Often, the craving will diminish within fifteen minutes.

Take Helpful Supplements

Some dietary supplements may help curb sugar cravings. Glutamic acid (the amino acid L-glutamine) has two major functions in the body. First, it fuels the brain—a feat matched by only one other compound, glucose. Second, glutamic acid restores hypoglycemic patients in insulin coma to consciousness at a lower blood sugar level than when glucose alone is used. L-glutamine might work to curb your sugar cravings. Take 500 milligrams three times a day.

Add chromium to your vitamin-mineral supplement. Sugar can deplete your body's chromium. Taking extra chromium can help to stabilize blood sugar. Add extra GTF (glucose tolerance factor) chromium to the vitamin-mineral supplement that you take for a total of 50 milligrams. Never take chromium or any other mineral alone as it can upset the delicate mineral balance in the body.

Avoid Soft Drinks

A glass of mineral water flavored with lemon, lime, or a tablespoon of orange or apple juice makes a great soft drink substitute. Sugar-free soft drinks are not acceptable substitutes; the phosphoric acid in all soft drinks changes the body's calcium-phosphorus ratio, upsetting its delicate chemical balance.

Keep Your Body in Homeostasis

It may take awhile for your unbalanced body to get back to homeostasis. Different organs can become oversensitive or underactive because of sugar abuse. It may take time for the organs to work properly again.

You can help by avoiding any foods to which you are allergic and by staying away from stressful situations. I recommend that you do not eat fruit until you have stopped having cravings. Fruit contains fructose and glucose, which will raise your blood sugar. For a sugar-sensitive person, fruit can change the mineral relationships. Coffee is another no-no. Coffee can lower your blood sugar, and you might experience such hypoglycemic symptoms as dizziness, lightheadedness, and perspiration, which can trigger a sugar craze. Alcohol is a stimulant to some and a depressant to others. Avoid any stimulant or depressant. The foods that help keep the body in homeostasis are vegetables, legumes, grains, and small amounts of protein.

Be Aware of Psychological Stressors

When you reach for that candy bar or soft drink, take a minute to look at your life and its stressors. Is there something that is making you anxious? Are you putting that sweet morsel in your mouth to soothe yourself? Try to make a connection between the stressors in your life and the need for "comfort food." Try to break the cycle.

Taste Sweetness Without Ingesting Sugar

Use fruit-flavored lip gloss. You can taste flavors such as apple, kiwi, melon, grape, mint, cantaloupe, and watermelon. Or brush your teeth. Most toothpastes contain a little sugar—not enough to do you any harm, but just enough to possibly satisfy your craving.

If your craving for sugar is very strong, put sugar, in whatever form, into your mouth, chew it, and then spit it out. This will give you the taste, but very little will get into your bloodstream. The best part is that you will be consciously rejecting the sugar by spitting it out.

Set Realistic Goals

You may not be able to cut out sugar all at once; phasing it out slowly may be a better plan. Set a date—a deadline for when you want to stop eating sugar altogether. Each day until that deadline, decrease your sugar intake by a given amount. If you slip, observe it, but don't wallow—move on. Set your goal again. Realize that even one day without sugar is a triumph.

When you finally do make your goal, reward yourself. Treat yourself to a professional massage, take yourself out to dinner, or enjoy some other special treat.

CONCLUSION

As your eating habits change, so will your taste buds.
Once you have successfully cut the sugar from your diet,
a carrot will taste as sweet as candy once did. Lightly
steamed carrots with a small amount of butter, which
were once something my mother made me eat, are now
a delicacy to me. You will begin to notice and appreciate
the natural sweetness in a number of healthful foods.

Chapter 11 offers a variety of recipes that promote
healthy eating while helping you curb the desire for
sugar.

11
Recipes

SOUPS

Garbure

1 cup dried navy or pea
  beans, soaked overnight
8 cups water
2 potatoes, sliced
2 onions, sliced
1–2 leeks, sliced
2 medium turnips, sliced
2 carrots, sliced
½ cup dried split peas
¼ cup minced fresh parsley

3 cloves garlic, minced
1 hot chili pepper
1 bay leaf
1 teaspoon thyme
1 teaspoon marjoram
½ small cabbage, shredded
½–1 pound roasted pork,
  chicken, goose, duck, beef, or
  other meat (optional)

Drain the beans and set aside. Bring the water to a boil in a large soup pot. Add the beans and all remaining ingredients except the cabbage and meat. Cover and bring quickly to a boil again. Reduce heat and simmer for 1 hour. Add the cabbage and roasted meat. Cover and bring quickly to a boil once more, then reduce heat and simmer for 30 minutes. Discard the bay leaf and chili pepper. Remove the meat, slice it, and place a serving in each bowl. Add soup. *Makes 4 to 6 servings.*

Hot Asparagus Soup

3 pounds asparagus, fresh or
   frozen
¼ pound butter
1 medium onion, chopped
6 cups chicken broth

½ teaspoon ground nutmeg
Salt to taste
Pepper to taste
2 tablespoons chopped fresh
   parsley or watercress

If using fresh asparagus, wash and remove the tough ends. Slice
the stalks into 2-inch pieces and set aside. Heat butter in a large,
heavy pot. Add onion and sauté until soft but not brown. Set aside
asparagus tips and add remaining asparagus pieces to pot. Cook 1
minute. Add broth, nutmeg, salt, and pepper. Bring to simmer and
cook until stalks are tender, about 18 minutes.

Add asparagus tips and cook until tender, about 3 minutes.
Remove some of the cooked tips and reserve for garnish. Purée
remaining cooked asparagus along with the cooking broth in a
blender 2 cups at a time. (Soup may be refrigerated at this point
and reheated when ready to serve.) Serve hot, garnished with
parsley and the reserved asparagus tips. *Makes 8 servings.*

Hearty Beet Borscht

3 large onions, chopped
3 beets, peeled and grated
2 potatoes, peeled and cubed
1 carrot, chopped
1 medium head red cabbage,
   shredded
2 quarts vegetable broth

2 fresh tomatoes, skinned and
   chopped
2 bay leaves, crumbled
1 tablespoon arrowroot
½ teaspoon dill
Salt to taste

In a large pot, combine all ingredients except salt. Simmer for
25 minutes. Add salt. *Makes 6 servings.*

Gingery Chicken Soup

1½ pounds chicken breasts
6 cups water
1½ teaspoons salt
3 tablespoons peeled, grated
  ginger root
3 green onions, sliced
  diagonally

1 cup sliced mushrooms
8½-ounce can water chestnuts,
  drained and diced
1 teaspoon soy sauce
1 cup shredded lettuce

Combine chicken, water, salt, and ginger in a large pot and bring to a boil. Reduce heat, cover, and simmer about 30 minutes or until chicken is tender. Turn off heat. Remove chicken and let cool slightly. Strain the broth, skimming any fat. Skin and bone the chicken, then cut it into ½-inch cubes. Heat broth to simmer. Add chicken, green onions, mushrooms, water chestnuts, and soy sauce. Simmer 10 minutes. Stir in lettuce just before serving. *Makes 6 servings.*

Vegetable Chowder

1 tablespoon safflower oil
1 medium onion, sliced
½ cup thinly sliced celery
1 clove garlic, minced
3 cups chicken broth
16-ounce can undrained
  tomatoes, chopped
1 cup sliced carrots

1 teaspoon dried basil
¼ teaspoon black pepper
1½ cups garbanzo beans
1½ cups fresh or frozen whole
  kernel corn
1 cup sliced zucchini

Heat oil in a large pot over medium-low heat. Add onion, celery, and garlic, and sauté until soft but not brown. Add broth, tomatoes, carrots, basil, and pepper. Cook about 25 minutes or until vegetables are tender. Add garbanzo beans, corn, and zucchini, and cook 5 more minutes. *Makes 8 servings.*

Manhattan Clam Chowder, Mexican Style

2 tablespoons safflower oil or
  butter
½ cup diced onion
½ cup diced celery
2 tablespoons arrowroot
1 cup chicken broth
12-ounce jar green chile salsa
½ cup diced potatoes
1 tablespoon minced fresh
  parsley

1 tablespoon chopped fresh
  basil
⅛ teaspoon thyme
½ bay leaf
Garlic powder to taste
Salt to taste
Pepper to taste
6-ounce can chopped clams

Heat oil in medium pot over low heat. Add onion and celery, and sauté until soft but not brown. Stir in arrowroot and continue to cook over low heat 2 minutes. Add chicken broth and simmer 3 minutes. Add salsa, potatoes, parsley, basil, thyme, bay leaf, garlic powder, salt and pepper. Simmer until potatoes are tender. Add clams and simmer an additional 5 minutes. *Makes about 4 servings.*

Broccoli Soup with Vegetables

1 cup broccoli florets
½ cup water
1½ cups chicken stock
½ cup fresh or frozen whole
  kernel corn

1 medium tomato, seeded and
  cut into thin wedges
Pepper to taste
⅛ teaspoon lemon juice

Place the broccoli on a steamer basket and set in a pot with the water. Steam the broccoli until just bright green. Remove the broccoli along with the basket and set aside. Add the chicken stock and corn to the water in the pot and simmer 5 minutes or until corn is almost tender. Add the tomatoes. Chop the broccoli, add it to the pot, and cook 5 minutes more. Add pepper and lemon juice. *Makes 4 servings.*

Spicy Bohemian-Style Tomato Soup

2 tablespoons butter
1 medium onion, chopped
2 stalks celery, chopped
2 quarts peeled and chopped
  fresh or canned tomatoes
1 quart vegetable stock

Salt to taste
Pepper to taste
1 heaping tablespoon mixed
  pickling spice (including
  bay leaf, chili pepper,
  ginger, and peppercorns)

Heat the butter in a large pot over medium-low heat. Add the onion and celery and sauté until soft but not brown. Add the tomatoes, stock, salt, and pepper. Bring to a boil. Place the pickling spice in a stainless steel tea ball and add to the soup. Simmer for 1 hour or until the tomatoes have cooked to a purée. *Makes 8 servings.*

Hot Borscht

1 cup tomato juice
1 cup beets, peeled and diced
1 parsnip, diced
2 cups potatoes, diced
1½ cups white cabbage, diced
1 tablespoon safflower oil
2 cloves garlic, minced

⅛ teaspoon vinegar
Salt to taste
Pepper to taste
Paprika to taste
Dill to taste
Parsley sprigs for garnish

In a blender, combine the tomato juice, beets, parsnip, potatoes, and white cabbage. Blend until smooth (add a little water, if necessary). Heat the oil in a medium pot over low heat. Add the garlic and sauté until soft but not brown. Add the blender mixture and vinegar to the pot and cook for 20 minutes. Season with salt, pepper, paprika, and dill. Ladle into soup bowls and top with parsley sprigs. *Makes 4 servings.*

VEGETABLES

Curried Peppers and Garbanzos

1 tablespoon butter or
safflower oil
1 clove garlic, finely minced
¼ cup chopped sweet onion
or scallion
1 medium green pepper,
thinly sliced
½ teaspoon dried basil

½ tablespoon chili powder
⅛ teaspoon cumin
⅛ coriander
⅛ dry mustard
Pepper to taste
1 cup vegetable juice cocktail
¾ cup cooked garbanzo beans

Heat butter in a medium skillet over medium-low heat. Add the garlic, onion, and green pepper and sauté until the vegetables are beginning to turn soft (do not brown). Season with basil, chili powder, cumin, coriander, mustard, and pepper. Add the vegetable juice cocktail and cook for about 5 minutes, allowing the flavors to blend. Add the garbanzo beans and continue to cook another 10 minutes. If mixture seems too thin, mash a few garbanzos with the back of a fork and blend to thicken. *Makes 4 small servings.*

Cabbage Scramble

½ cup tomato juice
½ teaspoon oregano
4 cups shredded cabbage
3 carrots, shredded

1 large onion, sliced and
separated into rings

Place all ingredients in a large skillet or pot. Cover and simmer over low heat 10 minutes, stirring often. Remove lid, turn up heat, and continue to stir until liquid is reduced. Serve hot. *Makes 4 to 6 servings.*

Fresh Potato Melange

¼ cup butter or safflower oil
2 large white potatoes, peeled and cut into julienne strips
1 large onion, chopped
1 large carrot, thinly sliced
2 celery stalks, sliced
1 clove garlic, chopped

2 cups chicken broth
1 bay leaf
¼ teaspoon crumbled dried thyme
Salt to taste
Pepper to taste

In large skillet, melt the butter over medium heat. Add the potatoes, onion, carrot, celery, and garlic, and sauté 2 to 3 minutes, stirring occasionally. Add the broth, bay leaf, thyme, salt, and pepper. Bring to a boil, cover, reduce heat, and simmer 10 minutes. Uncover, stir, and cook 5 minutes longer. With slotted spoon, remove vegetables to a serving bowl and cover to keep warm. Reduce cooking liquid over high heat until slightly thickened, about 2 minutes. Pour over vegetables. *Makes 4 servings.*

Barley-and-Corn-Stuffed Peppers

4 medium green bell peppers
¾ cup cooked barley
½ cup cooked corn
1 large tomato, skinned, seeded, and chopped
1 large scallion, chopped

2 tablespoons chopped fresh parsley
½ teaspoon dried basil
½ teaspoon chili powder
Salt to taste
Pepper to taste

Cut off tops from peppers. Remove the seeds and membranes, and steam the peppers for 5–6 minutes. Set aside and cool. To make the filling, combine the remaining ingredients in a large bowl. Stuff the peppers with the mixture and place in oiled casserole pan. Pour a half inch of water, stock, or tomato juice in the bottom of the pan. Bake at 350°F, covered, for 15 minutes. Remove cover and bake for 10 minutes more, adding more liquid if necessary. *Makes 4 servings.*

Savory Pepper Pilaf

2 tablespoons butter
1 clove garlic, minced
½ cup sweet onion, chopped
½ cup green pepper, chopped
1 cup cooked brown rice

Salt to taste
Pepper to taste
1 tablespoon Worcestershire
  sauce

Heat 1 tablespoon of the butter in a large skillet over medium-low heat. Add the garlic, onion, and green pepper, and sauté until they are just beginning to turn soft and are still crunchy. Add the remaining butter and the rice to the skillet. Season with salt and pepper. Combine the mixture well. Add the Worcestershire sauce and stir thoroughly. Cook 15 minutes. *Makes 2 servings.*

Ratatouille

¼ cup olive oil
4 cloves garlic, finely chopped
1 large onion, chopped
2 medium green peppers
2 small zucchini, cubed
2 small yellow squash, cubed
1 bunch parsley, chopped
4 tomatoes, skinned, seeded,
  and cubed

1 bay leaf
1 teaspoon chopped fresh basil
1 teaspoon marjoram
¼ teaspoon dried oregano
Salt to taste
Pepper to taste
2 cups prepared tomato purée

Heat the oil in a large pot over medium-low heat. Add the garlic and onion, and sauté until soft but not brown. Add the remaining ingredients and simmer until the vegetables are tender but not mushy. Serve over your favorite whole grain. *Makes 6 servings.*

Vegetarian Stew

1 tablespoon butter or
  safflower oil
2 cups thick-sliced fresh
  mushrooms
¼ cup chopped onion
1 clove garlic, finely minced
3–4 medium tomatoes,
  skinned, seeded, and cubed
1 medium zucchini, sliced

2 green peppers, seeded and
  cut into 1-inch chunks
1 tablespoon finely chopped
  fresh parsley
½ teaspoon chopped fresh
  basil
½ teaspoon marjoram
Salt to taste
Pepper to taste
¼ cup white wine (optional)

Melt the butter in a large skillet over medium-low heat. Add the mushrooms, onion, and garlic, and sauté until tender. Add all of the remaining ingredients except the wine. Simmer, covered, until vegetables are tender, about 15 minutes. Add the wine and continue to simmer another 5 minutes. *Makes 4 servings.*

Lentil Tomato Loaf

2 cups cooked lentils
2 cups tomato sauce
½ cup chopped onion
½ cup chopped celery
¾ cups oats

½ teaspoon garlic powder
¼ teaspoon Italian seasoning
¼ teaspoon celery seeds
Salt to taste
Pepper to taste

Combine all ingredients in a large bowl. Pack into an oiled 9-x-5-inch loaf pan. Bake at 350°F for 45 minutes. Let cool slightly before removing from pan. *Makes 4 servings.*

ENTRÉES

Persian Lamb and Bean Stew

⅔ cup dried kidney beans, white kidney beans (cannellini), Great Northern beans, or navy beans, soaked overnight and drained

7 cups water

5 tablespoons butter or safflower oil

1 pound coarsely chopped fresh spinach

⅓ pound) coarsely chopped fresh parsley

1 cup finely chopped leeks

¼ cup finely chopped green onions or scallions

1 tablespoon finely minced garlic

5 tablespoons olive oil

2 pounds lean lamb, cut into 1-inch cubes

2 tablespoons ground turmeric

2½ cups fresh or canned chicken broth

¼ cup fresh lemon juice

Salt to taste

Pepper to taste

Place the beans in a large pot or kettle along with the water and bring to a boil. Cover and cook until the beans are tender (from 30 minutes to 2 hours, depending on the type of bean). Do not overcook. When the beans are tender, remove from the heat, drain, and set aside.

Melt 3 tablespoons of the butter in the kettle over low heat. Add the spinach, parsley, leeks, green onions, and garlic. Cook, while stirring, until the greens are wilted. Set aside.

Heat the olive oil and remaining butter in a skillet. Cook the lamb, a few pieces at a time, until browned. (Do not crowd the skillet or the cubes will not brown properly.) As the cubes are cooked, transfer them to the kettle. Add the turmeric, chicken broth, and lemon juice to the kettle. Bring the ingredients to a boil, cover, and reduce the heat. Simmer about 1 hour or until the meat is almost fork-tender. Add the drained beans, salt, and pepper. Continue to simmer another 10–15 minutes. *Makes 8 servings.*

Spanish-Style Rice and Ground Beef

2 tablespoons safflower oil
2 medium onions, diced
1 medium green pepper,
  seeded and diced
¾ pound ground beef, cooked
  and drained
2 cups cooked brown rice

3 tomatoes, chopped
2 tablespoons lemon juice
½ cup tomato juice
½ teaspoon pepper
1 tablespoon onion powder
⅛ teaspoon garlic powder

Heat the oil in a large skillet over medium-low heat. Add the onion and green pepper, and sauté until soft. Add the remaining ingredients and combine well. Simmer 15 minutes. *Makes 4 servings.*

Irish Stew *

1 cup water
¾ cup cubed lamb (2-inch
  cubes)
¾ cup sliced onion
¾ cup sliced celery
½ cup sliced potatoes
½ cup sliced carrots

½ cup cut green beans
1 clove garlic, minced
1 small bay leaf
½ teaspoon dried mint
¼ teaspoon dried rosemary
¼ teaspoon dried marjoram
2 tablespoons arrowroot

Bring ½ cup of the water to a boil in a large pot over medium heat, and add all of the ingredients except the arrowroot. Reduce the heat to low and cook until the meat is tender, about 45 minutes. Mix the arrowroot with the remaining water and set aside. Move the vegetables to the sides of the pot, raise the heat to medium, and stir the arrowroot mixture into the broth. Continue to cook, while stirring, until the sauce is thick. Turn off heat and stir the vegetables gently into the sauce. Remove bay leaf. *Makes 2 servings.*

* From *The Candida Albicans Yeast-Free Cookbook.* Permission granted by the author, Pat Connolly, and Associates of the Price-Pottenger Nutrition Foundation, P.O. Box 2614, La Mesa, California.

SALADS AND SALAD DRESSINGS

Bulgarian Bean Salad

2 cups cooked navy beans or
  kidney beans
1 small green bell pepper,
  chopped
1 small sweet onion, chopped
1 large carrot, grated
¼ small head cabbage,
  shredded
2 tomatoes, chopped

Dressing:
  1 clove garlic, minced
  2 tablespoons chopped
    fresh parsley
  ½ cup safflower oil
  ¼ cup lemon juice
  Salt to taste
  Pepper to taste

In a large bowl, combine the beans and vegetables. Set aside.
Combine the dressing ingredients and pour over the salad. Toss to
coat thoroughly. Chill in refrigerator for 1 hour to blend flavors.
Serve on romaine lettuce. *Makes 2 to 3 servings.*

Basic Mayonnaise

2 eggs
1 teaspoon sea salt
¼ teaspoon dry mustard

¼ cup lemon juice
1¼ cups safflower oil (room
  temperature)

Place the eggs, salt, mustard, and lemon juice in a blender.
While blending, add the oil in a slow, steady stream, until mixture
is thick. Refrigerated and covered tightly, this mayonnaise will
keep up to one week. *Makes 1½ cups.*

Vegetable Rice Salad

4 cups cooked brown rice
1 cup bean or alfalfa sprouts
1 small zucchini, minced
1 small green bell pepper,
  minced
½ cup minced scallions
¼ cup minced fresh parsley

Dressing:
  ⅓ cup olive oil
  ¼ cup lemon juice
  ⅛ teaspoon cayenne
    pepper

In a salad bowl, toss together the rice, sprouts, zucchini, green pepper, scallions, and parsley. Combine the dressing ingredients and add to the rice mixture. Chill before serving. *Makes 4 to 6 servings.*

Molded Chicken Salad

3 cups cooked rice
2 cups chopped cooked
  chicken
1 cup cooked green peas
1 cup chopped celery
½ cup thinly sliced green
  onion including tops
1 avocado, peeled, pitted, and
  cubed

¼ cup chopped pimientos
2 envelopes unflavored gelatin
½ cup double-strength
  chicken broth (cold)
⅔ cup mayonnaise
1 tablespoon lemon juice
Salt to taste
Pepper to taste

In a large bowl, combine the rice, chicken, peas, celery, onion, avocado, and pimientos. In a small saucepan, add the gelatin to the broth, and heat to dissolve. Next, add the mayonnaise, lemon juice, salt, and pepper to the broth. Pour over the rice mixture and combine thoroughly. Spoon into a 1½-quart mold or individual molds. Chill to set. Remove the chilled salad from the mold and place on a bed of mixed salad greens. *Makes 6 to 8 servings.*

Broccoli and Potatoes Vinaigrette

2 medium-sized white
  potatoes
1½ cups broccoli florets
2 tablespoons chopped fresh
  parsley

Dressing:
1 clove garlic, finely minced
¼ teaspoon salt
2 tablespoons lemon juice
1 tablespoon water
Pepper to taste

Cut unpeeled potatoes into large cubes, and steam until they are half done when pierced with a knife. Add the broccoli florets to the potatoes and steam until the broccoli is tender-crisp and potatoes are completely cooked. Remove from the heat and set aside. To prepare the dressing, mash the garlic and salt together to form a paste. Add the lemon juice, water, and pepper, stirring it all together. If it is too sour, add more water. Pour the dressing over the vegetables. Sprinkle with fresh parsley and serve warm. *Makes 4 servings.*

Pepper Slaw

1 large green bell pepper,
  very thinly sliced
2 cups white cabbage,
  shredded
1 scallion, very thinly sliced

Dressing:
1 clove garlic, finely minced
¼ teaspoon salt
⅛ teaspoon dried basil
3 tablespoons lemon juice
Pepper to taste
¼ cup safflower oil

Toss bell pepper, cabbage, and scallion together in a bowl and set aside. To make the dressing, mash together the garlic and salt to form a smooth paste. Combine with the basil, lemon juice, and pepper. Beat in the oil with a fork. The dressing will begin to look cloudy and thicken slightly. Pour the dressing over the vegetables. Serve at room temperature or chilled. *Makes 4 servings.*

DESSERTS

The following sweet treats are made without sugar, fruit, fruit juice, or wheat. They are ideal when following Food Plan III.

Basic Pie Crust

⅓ cup barley flour　　　　　⅓ cup quinoa flour
⅓ cup rice flour　　　　　　½ cup melted butter

In a medium bowl, combine the flours. Using a fork, stir in the butter to form a dough. (If the dough is too dry, add a little water, a few drops at a time.) Form the dough into a ball and place between two pieces of wax paper. Roll out the dough into a 10-inch circle. Press the flattened dough into a 9-inch pie pan and crimp or flute the edges. Prick the bottom with a fork, and bake in a 450°F oven for 10 minutes or until light brown. Add your favorite "no-bake" filling to the cooked crust. (You can also add filling to the uncooked crust and bake according to individual recipe instructions.) *Makes one 9-inch single crust.*

Carob Mousse

6 cups well-cooked (baked or　　2 tablespoons vanilla
　steamed) sweet potatoes　　　½ cup powdered carob

Mix ingredients in a blender until thoroughly puréed. Pour into individual parfait glasses and refrigerate until ready to serve. *Makes 6 one-cup servings.*

This mousse can also be poured into a cooked Basic Pie Crust (see recipe above), refrigerated, and served.

Pumpkin Pie

2 pounds puréed fresh or
  canned pumpkin
4 eggs, beaten
2 teaspoons ground cinnamon

1 teaspoon ground ginger
½ teaspoon ground cloves
½ teaspoon ground nutmeg

Thoroughly mix ingredients together in a bowl. Pour into uncooked Basic Pie Crust (see page 197) and cook in preheated 450°F oven for 20 minutes or until a knife inserted in the center of the pie comes out clean.

To prepare without a crust, bake the filling in a 9-x-5-inch ovenproof baking dish or individual baking cups for 15 to 20 minutes, or until a knife inserted in the center of the filling comes out clean. *Serves 6 to 8.*

Coconut Sweet-Potato Pudding

4 cups well-cooked (baked or
  steamed) sweet potatoes
1 cup coconut milk

1 cup shredded fresh coconut
1 tablespoon vanilla

Mix ingredients in a blender until thoroughly puréed. Pour into individual parfait glasses and refrigerate until ready to serve. *Makes 6 one-cup servings.*

This pudding can also be poured into a cooked Basic Pie Crust (see page 197), refrigerated, and served.

Spicy Carob Brownies

1 cup quinoa flour
1 cup rice flour
1 cup powdered carob
2 teaspoons powdered ginger
1 rounded teaspoon cinnamon

2 teaspoons non-aluminum
baking powder
1 cup well-cooked (baked or
steamed) sweet potatoes
2 tablespoons safflower oil
2 eggs

Combine the quinoa flour, rice flour, carob, ginger, cinnamon, and baking powder in a bowl and set aside. In a large mixing bowl, beat together the sweet potatoes, oil, and eggs until well-blended. Add the dry ingredients to the sweet-potato mixture, about a half cup at a time, to form a smooth batter. Pour batter into a 7-x-11-inch greased and floured baking pan. Bake in a 350°F oven for 25 minutes or until a knife inserted in the center comes out clean. Allow to cool before cutting into squares and serving.

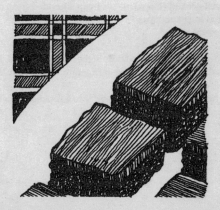

Epilogue

You have seen how your health can be jeopardized by eating excess sugar and a variety of other abusive substances, and by upsetting your body chemistry through stress and other bad habits. To summarize the chain of events: When the body is abused, its minerals become deficient. Since enzymes are dependent on minerals to function, they do not function optimally. This, in turn, causes incomplete digestion of food. Undigested food gets into the bloodstream. The cells cannot get the nutrients they need from the food in this undigested form. As a result, our immune system must come to our defense and escort this foreign protein (the undigested food) out of the body. The immune system, which was not meant to do this continually, becomes exhausted. The exhaustion of the immune system is the beginning of the degenerative disease process, which, depending on one's genetic blueprint, results in diseases or conditions such as arthritis and cancer.

I hope the information presented in this book is as

useful to you as it has been for me. Personally, it is exciting to know that I can maintain my own good health. I also feel a fulfillment in sharing what I have learned with others. And I can't help but wonder how much different my life might be today if I had had this information twenty years ago or, better yet, as I was growing up.

I was born with an endocrine system that secreted less than the ideal amount of some hormones and more of others. In itself, this may not have interfered with my quality of health or life. However, because of the stress I placed upon myself to excel as a child and the incredible amount of sugar I consumed, my body became less able to cope with abuse. Twenty years of my adult life were plagued with health problems.

Today I am in better health than I have been since I was eighteen years old. I need less sleep (six and a half hours instead of eight and a half), have more stamina, maintain an ideal weight, can consume an incredible amount of food, wake up happy, and go to bed happy every day. I feel good about myself and my relationships with others.

Now that I have taken responsibility for my health, I am not a victim of the twentieth-century lifestyle. I eat well, in spite of all the processed foods on supermarket shelves. I don't allow stress to become distress. I treat my body well. I am in control of my life and health. With a few simple, basic lifestyle changes, control can be yours also.

Glossary

Acute. Rapid; short; sudden; severe.

Adrenal gland. Either of two small endocrine glands, one located above each kidney. These glands consist of a cortex, which secretes several steroid hormones, and a medulla, which secretes adrenaline.

Adrenaline (epinephrine). One of the hormones secreted by the adrenal glands in response to physical or mental stress. Adrenaline initiates many bodily responses, including the stimulation of heart action and an increase in blood pressure, metabolic rate, and blood glucose concentration.

Allergen (antigen). A foreign protein, as in a food, bacteria, or virus, that stimulates a specific immune response when introduced into the body.

Amino acid. The end product of protein metabolism.

Anterior pituitary gland. *See* Pituitary gland.

Antibody. A protein substance produced in the blood that is capable of destroying or weakening bacteria or a toxin.

Antigen. *See* Allergen.

Biochemistry. The chemistry of live tissue.

Body chemistry. The functioning of the body's systems that depend upon chemical balance, which relies on balanced mineral relationships.

Carcinogen. Any substance that can cause cancer.

Cardiovascular. Relating to the heart and blood vessels.

Cataract. A cloudy film covering the lens of the eye that reduces the amount of incoming light.

Cholesterol. A chemical component of animal oils and fats. High amounts in the blood may be linked to the development of cholesterol deposits in the blood vessels (atherosclerosis).

Chronic. Pertaining to a disease or disorder that develops slowly and persists over a long period of time.

Chymotrypsin. An enzyme produced by the pancreas that aids in the digestion of milk proteins and gelatin in the small intestine.

Clinical ecologist. One who researches various causes of sickness that occur through exposure to substances such as food, manufactured chemicals, or pollutants.

Complement. Complex proteins in the blood that bind with substances (antibodies) that defend the body against foreign invaders (antigens). A deficiency or defect of any of the parts of a complement can occur. Those with complement abnormalities are more prone to infections.

Cytotoxic. Toxic to the cell.

Cytotoxic test. A blood test for food allergies.

Degeneration. Deterioration of normal cells and body functions.

Diabetes (mellitus). A chronic disease normally caused by the failure of the pancreas to release enough insulin into the bloodstream.

Endocrine system. A network of ductless glands—the pituitary, thyroid, parathyroid, and adrenals—that secrete hormones into the bloodstream.

Enzyme. A protein that acts as a biochemical catalyst to accelerate specific chemical reactions, but does not itself undergo any change during the reaction. Digestive enzymes break down complex carbohydrates into simple sugars; fats or lipids into fatty acids; and glycerol, glycerides, and protein into amino acids.

Epinephrine. *See* Adrenaline.

Estrogen. A group of steroid hormones that are formed in the ovaries, placenta, testes, and possibly the adrenal cortex. In addition to stimulation of secondary sexual characteristics, estrogen also exerts systemic effects such as growth and maturation of long bones.

Fatty acid. Any of several acids found in fats. An essential fatty acid (EFA) is one that cannot be produced by the body but is needed for the body's proper growth and functioning.

Free radical. An atom or molecule with an impaired electron. Free radicals are produced in the course of normal metabolism during the breakdown of oxidized fats in the body. They can also be produced by radiation, stress, food allergies, and other toxins.

Gastritis. Inflammation of the lining of the stomach.

Genetic blueprint. Inherited body chemistry.

Genetic potential. Inherited potential genetic blueprint.

Gland. An organ that manufactures a chemical to be utilized in the body. If this chemical is secreted into the bloodstream, the gland belongs to the endocrine system (e.g. thyroid, adrenals); if the secretion goes through a duct to surrounding tissue, it is an exocrine gland (e.g. sweat and salivary glands).

Glucose. A simple sugar, glucose is also called dextrose or grape sugar and is found in fruits, vegetables, tree sap, honey, corn syrup, and molasses. It is the end product of the digestion of starch, sucrose, maltose, and lactose, and provides most of the energy for the cells of the body.

Glycation. A condition in which sugar and protein are bound nonenzymatically in the body.

Glycogen. A major carbohydrate stored in the liver and muscles, glycogen is changed to glucose and released into the bloodstream as needed by the body for energy.

Glyconeogenesis. Glycogen synthesized by the liver from fats and proteins.

Gonad. Sex gland; the ovary or testicle.

HDL. *See* High-density lipoprotein.

Hemoglobin. Substance in the red blood cells that carries oxygen to the tissue.

High-density lipoprotein (HDL). A protein in blood plasma that carries cholesterol and other fats from the blood to the tissues.

Homeopathy. A branch of medicine that bases its system of treatment on the theory that "like cures like." Symptoms are treated with minute doses of plant, mineral, or animal substances that produce, in a healthy person, symptoms like those of the illness being treated.

Homeostasis (homeostatic mechanism). A mechanism used by the body to maintain a stable chemical internal environment, despite external change. This is accomplished in large part by the hormones.

Hormone. A chemical produced by a gland and secreted into the blood that affects the function of distant cells or organs.

Hydrochloric acid. Hydrogen chloride is an acid secreted by the cells lining the stomach. It aids in food digestion.

Hyper-. Prefix meaning "excessive," "above."

Hyperglycemia. A condition characterized by too much sugar in the blood, most often linked to diabetes mellitus.

Hypoglycemia. A condition characterized by too little sugar in the blood.

Hypothalamus. The master gland of the neuroendocrine system, the hypothalamus controls and integrates parts of the nervous system and endocrine processes, and many bodily functions such as temperature, sleep, and appetite.

Immune complex. Antigen combined with antibody. Tissue damage results when the complexes are formed in the presence of complement and leukocytes.

Immunoglobulins. Any of five families of antibodies in the serum and external secretions of the body. In response to certain antigens, immunoglobulins are formed in the bone marrow, spleen, and lymphoid body tissue (except the thymus).

In vitro. In glass; refers to experiments performed in test tubes rather than on living organisms.

Inflammation. A response of the body tissues to irritation or injury, inflammation is characterized by swelling, pain, increased temperature, and redness in the region of injury due to increased local blood flow.

Insulin. A hormone produced in the islets of Langerhans of the pancreas. When secreted into the bloodstream, insulin permits the metabolism and utilization of sugar.

Islets of Langerhans. The cells located in the pancreas that secrete insulin.

LDL. *See* Low-density lipoprotein.

Leukocyte. White blood cell.

Lipid. Fat.

Low-density lipoprotein (LDL). Portion of blood containing large amounts of cholesterol and triglycerides. LDLs are implicated in heart disease.

Menopause. The natural phase of a woman's life characterized by the cessation of menstruation.

Metabolic rate. The rate at which food is broken down in the body.

Metabolism. The process by which foods are transformed into basic elements that can be utilized by the body for energy or growth.

Mineral. An inorganic element, such as calcium, iron, potassium, sodium, and zinc, that is essential to the nutrition of humans, animals, and plants.

Naturopath. A practitioner who uses foods, supplements, water, and light in the treatment of illness.

Orthomolecular doctor. One who treats infectious and degenerative diseases by varying the concentration of substances, such as vitamins, minerals, trace elements, amino acids, enzymes, essential fatty acids, and hormones, which are normally present in the human body.

Osteoarthritis. A form of arthritis associated with bone and cartilage degeneration.

Osteoporosis. Loss of bone or skeletal tissue, producing brittleness or softness of bone.

Pancreas. A gland in upper portion of the abdomen that secretes insulin and glucagon into bloodstream, and digestive enzymes and bicarbonate into the intestine.

Parathyroid gland. One of four small endocrine glands located in the neck, the parathyroid secretes the hormone that controls calcium and phosphorus metabolism.

Pepsin. An enzyme secreted into the intestinal tract to aid in the digestion of food, particularly protein.

Periodontal disease. A disease of the tissues surrounding teeth.

pH. A scale denoting the acidity or alkalinity of a solution.

Phagocyte. A cell that can eat or destroy foreign matter or bacteria.

Pituitary gland. An endocrine gland located at the base of the brain, the pituitary secretes several hormones and controls the secretions of other glands such as the thyroid and adrenals. The anterior (front) portion of the pituitary produces many hormones including growth hormone. The posterior (back) portion of the pituitary secretes a number of hormones including an antidiuretic, which causes cells in the kidneys to absorb more water, thereby reducing the amount of urine.

Polypeptides. Intermediate state of protein breakdown. Polypeptides can do harm if they enter the bloodstream before they are broken down into amino acids.

Postpituitary gland (posterior pituitary). *See* Pituitary gland.

Postprandial. Following a meal.

Progesterone. A steroid hormone secreted primarily by ovaries and placenta, progesterone stimulates secretion by uterine glands, inhibits contraction of uterine smooth muscle, and stimulates breast growth.

Prostaglandins. A group of fatty acids that function as chemical messengers, made in most, possibly all, cells of the body. Protaglandins transmit chemical signals between cells or between one area of a cell and another area.

Rarefy. To make or become thin or less dense.

Rheumatoid arthritis. A long-term connective tissue disease characterized by inflammation of the synovial membranes that line the joints. This leads to thickness of the synovial membrane and joint swelling, which results in pain and limitation of motion.

Thyroid. Endocrine gland located in front of the neck that regulates body metabolism. The thyroid secretes thyroxin, which is essential to normal body growth in infancy and childbirth.

Thyroxin. The hormone manufactured by the thyroid gland, essential for normal body growth in infants and children.

Triglycerides. This class of fats makes up most animal and vegetable fats and appears in the blood bound to a protein, forming
high- and low-density lipoproteins.

Victim. Not known in this book.

Notes

Chapter 1

1. Arthur F. Coca. *The Pulse Test.* (New York: Arco Publishing Company, 1978.)
2. Beatrice Trum Hunter. "Confusing Consumers About Sugar Intake," *Consumer's Research* 78, No. 1, January 1995.
3. "United States Sugar Policy: An Analysis." (Washington, DC: U.S. Printing Office, 1989, p. 4).
4. Melvin Page. *Body Chemistry in Health and Disease.* (La Mesa, CA: Price-Pottenger Nutrition Foundation, circa 1954.)

Inset: Sugar-Coating the Truth

1. George McGovern, Edward M. Kennedy, Hubert H. Humphrey, Alan Cranston, Robert Dole, et al. *Dietary Goals for the United States.* (Washington DC: United States Printing Office, 1977.)
2. Walter H. Glinsmann, Hiltje Irausquin, and Youngmee Park. *Report from FDA's Sugars Task Force 1986: Evaluation of Health Aspects of Sugars Contained in Carbohydrate Sweeteners.* (Washington, DC: Center for Food Safety and Applied Nutrition, 1986, p. 39.)
3. "Estimated Annual Production and Consumption of Soft Drinks." Washington, DC, Soft Drink Association, 1987.
4. University of California Berkeley, *Berkeley Wellness Letter* 6, No. 3, December 1989, pp. 4–5.

Chapter 2

1. Jeffrey Bland. *Digestive Enzymes.* (New Canaan, CT: Keats Publishing, 1983.)
2. Melvin Page, and H. Leon Abram, Jr. *Your Body is Your Best Doctor.* (New Canaan, CT: Keats Publishing, 1972.)
3. J. Lemann. "Evidence that Glucose Ingestion Inhibits Net Renal Tubular Reabsorption of Calcium and Magne-

sium," *Journal of Clinical Nutrition* 70, 1967, pp. 236–245.

4. Walter B. Cannon. *The Wisdom of the Body.* (New York: Norton and Company, 1963.)

5. Melvin Page, and H. Leon Abram, Jr. *Your Body is Your Best Doctor.* (New Canaan, CT: Keats Publishing, 1972.)

6. David L. Watts. "Nutrient Interrelationships: Minerals - Vitamins - Endocrines," *Journal of Orthomolecular Medicine* 5, No. 1, 1990, pp. 11–19.

7. E. Planells, et al. "Changes in Bioavailability and Tissue Distribution of Zinc Caused by Magnesium Deficiency in Rats," *British Journal of Nutrition* 72, August 1994, pp. 315–323.

8. Melvin Page. *Body Chemistry in Health and Disease.* (La Mesa, CA: Price-Pottenger Nutrition Foundation, circa 1954.)

9. Carlson Wade. *Helping Your Health with Enzymes.* (New York: ARC Books, 1971.)

Chapter 3

1. Theron G. Randolph, and Leona B. Yeager. "Corn Sugar as an Allergen." *Annals of Allergy,* September–October, 1949, pp. 650–661.

2. Joel Wallach. "Metabolic Therapy." Paper presented at the National Health Federation Meeting, Long Beach, CA, January 1983. Audio tape.

3. George A. Ulett. "Food Allergy—Cytotoxic Testing and the Central Nervous System." *Psychiatric Journal of the University of Ottawa* 5, No. 2, June 1980, pp. 100–108.

4. Joel Wallach. "Metabolic Therapy for Heart Disease, Cancer, Allergies, and Multiple Sclerosis." Paper presented at the National Health Federation Meeting, Long Beach, CA, January, 1983. Audio tape.

5. Arthur L. Kaslow, and Richard B. Miles. *Freedom from Chronic Disease.* (Los Angeles: J.P. Tarcher, 1979.)

6. Leonard Bjeldanes. "Effect of Over-Cooked Meat." *Journal of Food and Chemical Toxicology* 23, No. 12, April 1985.

7. H. Harrow Brown. "The Diagnosis and Management of Allergy." From paper delivered at the annual meeting of the Indian College of Allergy and Immunology, Simla, AZ, September 1980.

8. K. Willeke, and K. Whitley. "Aerosols: Size Distribution Interpretation." *Air Pollution Control Association Journal* 25, No. 526, p. 196.

9. Amelia Nathan Hill. Amelia Nathan Hill International Foundation of Collating Al-

lergy Research, Wimbledon, England, April 4, 1983. Personal interview.

10. William Rea, et al. "Food and Chemical Susceptibility After Environmental Chemical Overexposure: Case Histories." *Annals of Allergy* 41, August 1978, pp. 101–110.

Chapter 4

1. Hans Selye. *The Stress of Life*. (San Francisco, CA: McGraw-Hill, 1978.)
2. Ibid.
3. William H. Philpott, and Dwight K. Kalita. *Brain Allergies*. (New Canaan, CT: Keats Publishing, 1980.)
4. Ibid.
5. Ibid.
6. W. Ringsdorf, E. Cheraskin, and E. Ramsey. "Sucrose Neutrophilic Phagocytosis and Resistance to Disease." *Dental Survey* 52, No. 12, 1976, pp. 46–48.
7. A. Sanchez, et al. "Role of Sugars in Human Neutrophilic Phagocytosis." *American Journal of Clinical Nutrition*, November 1973, pp. 1180–1184.
8. Ernest Kijak, George Foust, and Ralph Steinman. "Relationship of Blood Sugar Level and Leukocytic Phagocy-

tosis." *Southern California State Dental Association Journal* 32, No. 8, September 1964.

9. F. Bunn, and P.J. Higgins. "Reaction of Monosaccharides with Protein: Possible Evolutionary Significance." *Science* 213, July 10, 1981, pp. 222–224.

10. R. Pamplona, M.J. Bellmunt, M. Portero, and J. Prat. "Mechanisms of Glycation in Atherogenesis," *Medical Hypotheses* 40, 1990, pp. 174–181.

11. Anna Furth, and John Harding. "Why Sugar is Bad for You," *New Scientist*, September 23, 1989, p. 44.

12. "Estimated Annual Production and Consumption of Soft Drinks." Washington, DC: Soft Drink Association, 1986.

Chapter 5

1. Glen W. King. *Statistical Abstracts of the U.S.* (Washington, DC: U.S. Government Printing Office, 1993, p. 85.)
2. *Historical Statistics of the U.S.—Colonial Times to 1970*. (Washington, DC: U.S. Government Printing Office, 1975, p. 65.)
3. Brian W. Morris, et al. "Trace Element Chromium—A Role in Glucose Homeostasis." *American Journal of Clinical*

Nutrition 55, 1992, pp. 989–991.

4. Derrick Lonsdale. "A Sugar Sensitive Athlete: Case Report." *Journal of Advancement in Medicine* 7, No. 1, Spring 1994, pp. 51–58.

5. William H. Philpott, and Dwight K. Kalita. *Victory over Diabetes*. (New Canaan, CT: Keats Publishing, 1983.)

6. James F. Balch, and Phyllis A. Balch. *Prescription for Nutritional Healing*. (Garden City Park, NY: Avery Publishing Group, 1996.)

7. Ibid.

8. A. Kozlovsky, et al. "Effects of Diets High in Simple Sugars on Urinary Chromium Losses." *Metabolism* 35, June 1986, pp. 515–518.

9. William H. Philpott, and Dwight K. Kalita. *Victory over Diabetes*. (New Canaan, CT: Keats Publishing, 1983.)

10. H. Keen, B. Thomas, R. Jarrett, and L. Fuller. "Nutritional Intake, Adiposity, and Diabetes." *British Medical Journal* 1, 1989, pp. 655–658.

11. Mark Nathan Cohn. *The Rise of Civilization*. (New Haven, CT: Yale University Press, 1989.)

12. Rebecca Buckley. "Food Allergy." *Journal of the American Medical Association* 248, 1982, pp. 26–27.

13. Roger C. Wiggins, and M.P. Cochrane. "Immune Complex—Medicated Biological Effects." *New England Journal of Medicine* 304, 1981, p. 518.

14. William E. Catterall. "Rheumatoid Arthritis Is an Allergy." *Arthritis News Today*, 1980.

15. L.G. Darlington, N.W. Ramsey, and J.R. Mansfield. "Placebo-Controlled, Blind Study of Dietary Manipulation Therapy in Rheumatoid Arthritis." *Lancet*, February 6, 1986, pp. 236–238.

16. James F. Balch, and Phyllis A. Balch. *Prescription for Nutritional Healing*. (Garden City Park, NY: Avery Publishing Group, 1996.)

17. Lawrence Power. "Sensitivity: You React to What You Eat." *Los Angeles Times*, February 12, 1985.

18. A.H. Rowe, and E.J. Young. "Bronchial Asthma Due To Food Allergy Alone in Ninety-five Patients." *Journal of the American Medical Association* 169, 1959, p. 1158.

19. Sandra Blakeslee. "Despite Improved Drugs, Death Rate from Asthma Doubles in a Decade." *The New York Times*, March 24, 1988, Health section, p. 18.

20. Lawrence Power. "Special Diets Ease Some Headache

Pain." *Los Angeles Times*, August 12, 1984.

21. J. Egger, et al. "Is Migraine Food Allergy?" *Lancet*, October 15, 1983, pp. 865–867.

22. Ellen Grant. "Food Allergy and Migraine." *Lancet* 8123, 1979, pp. 966–969.

23. W.K. Amery, and P.P. Forget. "The Role of the Gut in Migraine: The Oral 51-Cr EDTA Test in Recurrent Abdominal Pain." *Cephalaquia* 9, 1989, pp. 227–229.

24. John M. Douglass. "Psoriasis and Diet." *Western Journal of Medicine* 133, November 1980, p. 450.

25. Matthew Van Dolde. *Biochemistry*. (Redwood City, CA: Benjamin Cummings Publishing Company, 1990, p. 186.)

26. Clara J. Moerman, H. Bas Bueno De Mesquita, and Sylske Runia. "Dietary Sugar Intake in the Etiology of Biliary Tract Cancer." *International Journal of Epidemiology* 22, 1993, pp. 207–214.

27. Donald B. Pribor. *Overview of Physiological Stability*. (Dubuque, IA: Kendall/Hunt, 1987.)

28. Herta Spencer, and Lois Kramer. "Antacid-Induced Calcium Loss." *Archives of Internal Medicine* 143, No. 4, April 1983, pp. 657–659.

29. D.P. Kiel, David T. Felson, Marian T. Hannan, Jennifer Anderson, and Peter W. Wilson. "Caffeine and the Risks of Hip Fracture: The Framingham Study." *American Journal of Epidemiology* 132, No. 4, October 1990, pp. 675–684.

30. J.J. Michnoviez, R.J. Hershcopf, H. Naganuna, et al. "Increased 2-Hydroxylation of Oestradoil as a Possible Mechanism for the Anti-Oestrogenic Effect of Cigarette Smoking." *New England Journal of Medicine* 35, 1986, pp. 1305–1309.

31. L.H. Allen. "Calcium Absorption and Bioavailability: A Review." *American Journal of Clinical Nutrition* 35, 1983, pp. 783–808.

32. R. Itoh, et al. "Salt Increases Calcium Loss." *The Nutrition Report* 10, No. 3, March 1992, p. 20.

33. C. Cooper, et al. "Water Fluoridation and Hip Fracture." *Journal of the American Medical Society* 19, No. 32, July 1991, pp. 513–514.

34. D.D. Saville. "Changes in Bone Mass with Age and Alcoholism." *Journal of Bone and Joint Surgery* 47A, 1965, p. 492.

35. J.A. Thom, et al. "The Influence of Refined Carbohydrates on Urinary Calcium

Excretion." *British Journal of Urology* 50, No. 7, December 1987, pp. 459–464.

36. "Calcium for Osteoporosis, Little Help, Little Harm." *Family Practice News*, February 15, 1994, p. 14.

37. L.H. Allen, G.D. Block, R.N. Wood, and G.F. Bryce. "The Role of Insulin and Parathyroid Hormone in the Protein-Induced Calciuria of Man." *Nutrition Research* 1, 1981, p. 11.

38. J. Ayalon, A. Simkin, I. Leichter, and S. Raefmann. "Dynamic Bone Loading Exercise of Postmenopausal Women." *Archives of Physical Rehabilitation* 68, No. 5, May 1987, pp. 280–283.

39. T. David, et al. "The Effect of Postmenopausal Estrogen Therapy on Bone Density in Elderly Women." *New England Journal of Medicine* 329, No. 16, October 14, 1993, pp. 1141–1146.

40. Miles H. Robinson. "On Sugar and White Flour—The Dangerous Twins." In *A Physician's Handbook to Orthomolecular Medicine*. Roger William and Dwight K. Kalita, eds. (New York: Pergamon Press, 1978, pp. 24–28.)

41. John Yudkin. "Dietary Fat and Dietary Sugar in Relation to Ischemic Heart Disease and Diabetes." *Lancet* 2, No. 4, 1964.

42. WIlliam H. Philpott, and Dwight K. Kalita. *Victory over Diabetes*. (New Canaan, CT: Keats Publishing, 1983.)

43. John Yudkin. "Dietary Fat and Dietary Sugar in Relation to Ischemic Heart Disease and Diabetes." *Lancet* 2, No. 4, 1964.

44. J. Raloff. "Oxydized Lipids: A Key to Heart Disease." *Science News* 127, May 2, 1985, p. 278.

45. Ibid.

46. Hans Selye. *Stress Without Distress*. (Philadelphia: Lippincot, Inc., 1974.)

47. R.J. Doisy. *Minerals and Trace Elements*. pp. 586–594.

48. William H. Philpott, and Dwight K. Kalita. *Victory over Diabetes*. (New Canaan, CT: Keats Publishing, 1983.)

49. J.M. McKenzie. "Urinary Excretion of Cadmium, Zinc and Copper in Normotensive and Hypertensive Women." *New England Medical Journal* 78, July 1973, pp. 68–70.

50. J. Hallfrisch, et al. "The Effects of Fructose on Blood Lipid Levels." *American Journal of Clinical Nutrition* 37, No. 5, 1983, pp. 740–748.

51. Frances Sheridan Goulart. "Behind Bars, Kicking the

Candy Bar Habit," parts 1 and 2. *Herbalist New Health,* January and February 1981.

52. R.J. Kuczmarski, et al. "Increased Prevalence of Overweight U.S. Adults." *Journal of the American Medical Association* 272, July 20, 1994, pp. 205–211.

53. Thomas A. Wadden, et al. "Responsible and Irresponsible Use of Very-Low-Calorie Diets in the Treatment of Obesity." *Journal of the American Medical Association* 263, No. 1, January 5, 1990, pp. 83–86.

54. Torbjorn Backstrom, and Serfan Hammerback. "Premenstrual Syndrome—Psychiatric or Gynecological Disorder." *Annals of Medicine* 23, 1991, pp. 625–633.

55. Katherine Dalton. "Diet of Women with Severe Premenstrual Syndrome and the Effects of Changing to a Three-Hour Starch Diet." *Stress Medicine* 81, 1992, pp. 61–65.

56. Annette MacKay Rossignol. "Prevalence and Severity of Premenstrual Syndrome: Effects of Food and Beverages That are Sweet or High in Sugar Content." *The Journal of Reproductive Medicine* 36, No. 2, February 1991, pp. 131–136.

57. Marilyn Hamilton Light. "Premenstrual Tension." *Homeostasis Quarterly,* Adrenal Metabolic Research Society of the Hypoglycemia Foundation, March 1984.

58. James F. Balch, and Phyllis A. Balch. *Prescription for Nutritional Healing.* (Garden City Park, NY: Avery Publishing Group, 1996.)

59. C. Orion Truss. *The Missing Diagnosis.* (Birmingham, AL: C. Truss, 1983.]

60. C. Orion Truss. "Restoration of Immunologic Competence to Candida Albicans." *Orthomolecular Psychiatry* 9, No. 4, 1980, pp. 287–301.

61. James F. Balch, and Phyllis A. Balch. *Prescription for Nutritional Healing.* (Garden City Park, NY: Avery Publishing Group, 1996.)

62. Shirley Lorenzani. "Candida Albicans." Audio cassette tapes, set I and II. (La Mesa, CA: Price-Pottenger Nutrition Foundation, circa 1980.)

63. William G. Crook. *The Yeast Connection.* (Jackson, TN: Professional Books, 1984.)

64. DeWayne Ashmead. *Chelated Mineral Nutrition.* (Huntington Beach, CA: Institute Publishers, 1981.)

65. Ralph Steinman. Loma Linda University unpublished research on the effects of sugar on tooth decay. In-

formation obtained through communication with Bruce Pacetti, DDS.

66. D. Gay, G. Dick, and G. Upton. "Multiple Sclerosis Associated with Sinusitis: Case-Controlled Study in General Practice." *Lancet* 8940, No. 1, April 1986, pp. 815–819.

67. Arthur L. Kaslow, and Richard B. Miles. *Freedom from Chronic Disease.* (Los Angeles: J.P. Tarcher, 1979.)

68. Linda Garmon. "Crohn's Disease: Intestinal Enigma." *Science News* 177, May 3, 1980, pp. 280–281.

69 .V.A. Jones, et al. "Food Intolerance: A Major Factor in the Pathogenesis of Irritable Bowel Syndrome." *Lancet*, November 10, 1982, pp. 1115–1117.

V.A. Jones, et al. "Crohn's Disease: Maintenance of Remission by Diet." *Lancet*, July 27, 1985, pp. 177–180.

D.J. Pearson, K. Rix, and S. Bently. "Food Allergy: How Much in the Mind." *Lancet* 2, 1983, pp. 1259–1261.

M. Petitpierre, P. Guimowski, and J.P. Girard. "Irritable Bowel Syndrome and Hypersensitivity to Food." *Annals of Allergy* 54, June 1985, pp. 538–540.

70. James F. Balch, and Phyllis A. Balch. *Prescription for Nutritional Healing.* (Garden City Park, NY: Avery Publishing Group, 1996.)

71. Lawrence Power. "Change in Diet May Help Relieve Asthma Patient." *Los Angeles Times*, May 7, 1985.

72. *The Signet/Mosby Medical Encyclopedia*, (New York: Penguin Books, 1987.)

73. Jack Joseph Challem, and Renate Lewin. "Vitamins and Fiber for Preventing Gallstones." *Let's Live*, April 14, 1984, pp. 10–12.

74. Jack Joseph Challem, and Renate Lewin. "Vitamins and Fiber for Preventing Gallstones." *Let's Live*, April 14, 1984, pp. 10–12.

75. K.W. Heaton. "The Sweet Road to Gallstones." *British Medical Journal* 288, April 14, 1984, pp. 1103–1104.

76. Burton Goldburg Group. *Alternative Medicine.* (Payallup, WA: Future Medicine Publishing, Inc., 1993, pp. 942–943.)

77. O.M. Embon, et al. "Chronic Dehydration Stone Disease." *British Journal of Urology* 66, 1990, pp. 357–362.

78. G.C. Curran, et al. "A Prospective Study of Dietary Calcium and Other Nutrients and the Risk of Symptomatic Kidney Stones." *New England Journal of Medicine*

328, No. 12, March 25, 1993, pp. 833–838.

79. J.M. Braganza. "Selenium Deficiency, Cystic Fibrosis, and Pancreatic Cancer." *Lancet* 2, 1986, p. 1238.

R.J. Stead, et al. "Selenium Deficiency and Possible Increased Risk of Carcinoma in Adults with Cystic Fibrosis." *Lancet* 2, 1986, p. 862.

80. J.D. Wallach, and B. Germaise. "Cystic Fibrosis: A Perinatal Manifestation of Selenium Deficiency." *Trace Substances in Environmental Health.*" D.D. Hemphill, ed. (Colombia, MO: University of Missouri Press, 1979.)

81. Francis M. Pottenger, Jr. *Pottenger's Cats.* (La Mesa, CA: Price-Pottenger Nutrition Foundation, 1979.)

Inset: How Sugar and Sweeteners Can Ruin Your Health

1. A. Sanchez, et al. "Role of Sugars in Human Neutrophilic Phagocytosis." *American Journal of Clinical Nutrition*, November 1973, pp. 1180–1184.

2. F. Couizy, C. Keen, M.E. Gershwin, and F.P. Mareschi. "Nutritional Implications of the Interaction Between Minerals." *Progressive Food and Nutrition Science* 17, 1933, pp.65–87.

3. J. Goldman, et al. "Behavioral Effects of Sucrose on Preschool Children." *Journal of Abnormal Child Psychology* 14, No. 4, 1986, pp. 565–577.

4. D. Behar, J. Rapoport, Berg C. Adams, and M. Cornblat. "Sugar Testing with Children Considered Behaviorally Sugar Reactive." *Nutritional Behavior* 1, 1984, pp. 277–288.

5. Alexander Schauss. *Diet, Crime and Delinquency.* (Berkeley, CA: Parker House, 1981.)

6. S. Scanto, and John Yudkin. "The Effect of Dietary Sucrose on Blood Lipids, Serum Insulin, Platelet Adhesiveness and Body Weight in Human Volunteers." *Postgraduate Medicine Journal* 45, 1969, pp. 602–607.

7. W. Ringsdorf, E. Cheraskin, and R. Ramsay. "Sucrose Neutrophilic Phagocytosis and Resistance to Disease." *Dental Survey* 52, No. 12, 1976, pp. 46–48.

8. J. Yudkin, S. Kang, and K. Bruckdorfer. "Effects of High Dietary Sugar." *British Journal of Medicine* 281, November 22, 1980, p. 1396.

9. Ibid.

10. R. Pamplona, M.J. Bellmunt,

M. Portero, and J. Prat. "Mechanisms of Glycation in Atherogenesis." *Medical Hypotheses* 40, 1990, pp. 174–181.

11. A. Kozlovsky, et al. "Effects of Diets High in Simple Sugars on Urinary Chromium Losses." *Metabolism* 35, June 1986, pp. 515–518.

12. M. Fields, et al. "Effect of Copper Deficiency on Metabolism and Mortality in Rats Fed Sucrose or Starch Diets." *Journal of Clinical Nutrition* 113, 1983, pp. 1335–1345.

13. "Sugar and Prostate Cancer." *Health Express*, October, 1982, p. 41.

14. R.M. Bostick, J.D. Potter, L.H. Kushi, et al. "Sugar, Meat, and Fat Intake, and Non-dietary Risk Factors for Colon Cancer Incidence in Iowa Women." *Cancer Causes and Controls* 5, 1994, pp. 38–52.

15. Clara Moerman, et al. "Dietary Sugar Intake in the Etiology of Biliary Tract Cancer." *International Journal of Epidemiology* 22, No. 2, 1993, pp. 207–214.

16. J. Kelsay, et al. "Diets High in Glucose or Sucrose and Young Women." *American Journal of Clinical Nutrition* 27, 1974, pp. 926–936.

17. J. Lemann. "Evidence That Glucose Ingestion Inhibits Net Renal Tubular Reabsorption of Calcium and Magnesium." *Journal of Clinical Nutrition* 70, 1967, pp. 236–245.

18. H. Ed Taub, ed. "Sugar Weakens Eyesight." *VM Newsletter* 5, May 1986.

19. Richard Wurtman. *University of California, Berkeley, Newsletter* 6, No. 3, December 1989, pp. 4–5.

20. William Dufty. *Sugar Blues.* (New York: Warner Books, 1975.)

21. Ibid.

22. J. Lewis. "Health Briefings." *Fort Worth Star Telegram*, June 11, 1990.

23. Timothy Jones. "Health Briefings." *Fort Worth Star Telegram*, June 11, 1990.

24. Annette T. Lee, and Anthony Cerami. "The Role of Glycation in Aging." *Annals of the New York Academy of Science* 663, pp. 63–70.

     D.G. Dyer, et al. "Accumulation of Maillard Reaction Products in Skin Collagen in Diabetes and Aging." *Journal of Clinical Investigation* 91, No. 6, June 1993, pp. 421–422.

25. E. Abrahamson, and A. Peget. *Body, Mind and Sugar.* (New York: Avon, 1977.)

26. W. Glinsmann, H. Irausquin, and K. Youngmee. *Report from*

FDA's *Sugar Task Force, 1986: Evaluation of Health Aspects of Sugars Contained in Carbohydrate Sweeteners.* (Washington, DC: Center for Food Safety and Applied Nutrition, 1986, p. 39.)

27. H. Keen, B. Thomas, R. Jarrett, and J. Fuller. "Nutrient Intake, Adiposity, and Diabetes." *British Medical Journal* 6164, No. 1, March 10, 1979, pp. 655–658.

28. T. Cleave. *Sweet and Dangerous.* (New York: Bantam Books, 1974, pp. 28–43.)

    B.G. Persson, et al. "Diet and Inflammatory Bowel Disease." *Epidemiology* 3, No. 1, January 1992, pp. 47–51.

29. T. Cleave. *Sweet and Dangerous.* (New York: Bantam Books, 1974, pp. 157–159.)

30. L. Darlington, Ramsey, and Mansfield. "Placebo-Controlled, Blind Study of Dietary Manipulation Therapy in Rheumatoid Arthritis." *Lancet* 8475, No. 1, February 6, 1986, pp. 236–238.

31. Lawrence Powers. "Sensitivity: You React to What You Eat." *Los Angeles Times*, February 12, 1985.

32. W. Crook. The Yeast Connection. (Jackson, TN: Professional Books, 1984.)

33. K. Heaton. "The Sweet Road to Gallstones." *British Medical Journal* 288, April 14, 1984, pp. 1103–1104.

34. N.J. Blacklock. "Sucrose and Idiopathic Renal Stone." *Nutrition and Health* 5, No. 1–2, 1987, pp. 9–17.

35. J. Yudkin. "Dietary Fat and Dietary Sugar." *Lancet*, August 29, 1964, pp. 478–479.

36. T. Cleave. *The Saccharine Disease.* (New Canaan, CT: Keats Publishing, 1974, p. 125.)

37. S. Erlander. "The Cause and Cure of Multiple Sclerosis." *The Disease to End Disease* 1, No. 3, March 3, 1979, pp. 59–63.

38. T. Cleave. *The Saccharine Disease.* (New Canaan, CT: Keats Publishing, 1974, p. 45.)

39. T. Cleave, and G. Campbell. *Diabetes, Coronary Thrombosis and the Saccharine Disease.* (Bristol, England: John Wright and Sons, 1960.)

40. K. Behall. "Influence of Estrogen Content of Oral Contraceptives and Consumption of Sucrose on Blood Parameters." *Disease Abstracts International B.* 43, 1982, p. 1437.

41. W. Glinsmann, H. Irausquin, and K. Youngmee. *Report from FDA's Sugar Task Force, 1986: Evaluation of Health Aspects of Sugars Contained in Carbohydrate Sweeteners.* (Washington, DC: Center for Food

Safety and Applied Nutrition, 1986, p. 39.)

42. Nancy Appleton. *Healthy Bones.* (Garden City Park, NY: Avery Publishing Group, 1989, pp. 36–38.)

43. Ibid.

44. H. Beck-Nelson., O. Pedersen, and Sorensen Schwartz. "Effects of Diet on the Cellular Insulin Binding and the Insulin Sensitivity in Young Healthy Subjects." *Diabetes* 15, 1978, pp. 289–296.

45. H. Keen, B. Thomas, R. Jarrett, and J. Fuller. "Nutritional Factors in Diabetes Mellitus." J. Yudkin, ed. *Applied Science*, 1977, pp. 89–108.

46. L. Gardner, and S. Reiser. "Effects of Dietary Carbohydrate on Fasting Levels of Human Growth Hormone and Cortisol." *Proceedings of the Society for Experimental Biology and Medicine* 169, 1982, pp. 36–40.

47. S. Reiser. "Effects of Dietary Sugars on Metabolic Risk Factors Associated with Heart Disease." *Nutritional Health* 3, 1985, pp. 203–216.

48. R. Hodges, and T. Rebello. "Carbohydrates and Blood Pressure." *Annals of Internal Medicine* 98, 1983, pp. 838–841.

49. J. Simmons. "Is the Sand of Time Sugar?" *Longevity*, June 1990, pp. 49–53.

F. Bunn, and P.J. Higgins. "Reaction of Monosaccharides with Protein: Possible Evolutionary Significance." *Science* 213, July 10, 1981, pp. 222–224.

Anthony Cerami, Helen Vlassara, and Michael Brownlee. "Glucose and Aging." *Scientific American*, May 1987, p. 90.

50. Nancy Appleton. *Healthy Bones.* (Garden City Park, NY: Avery Publishing Group, 1991.)

51. "Sucrose Induces Diabetes in Cats." *Federal Protocol* 6, No. 97, 1974.

52. T. Cleave. *The Saccharine Disease.* (New Canaan, CT: Keats Publishing, 1974, pp. 132–133.)

53. Ibid.

54. Ruth L. Caccaro, and J. Stamle. "Relationship of Postload Plasma Glucose to Mortality with a Follow-Up." *Diabetic Care* 15, No. 10, October 1992.

55. Annette T. Lee, and Anthony Cerami. "Modifications of Proteins and Nucleic Acids by Reducing Sugars: Possible Role in Aging." *Handbook of the Biology of Aging.* (New York: Academic Press, 1990.)

56. Suresh I.S. Rattan, Anastasia

Derventzi, and Brian Clark. "Protein Synthesis, Post-translational Modifications, and Aging." *Annals of the New York Academy of Sciences* 663, 1992, pp. 48–62.

57. V.M. Monnier. "Nonenzymatic Glycosylation, the Maillard Reaction and the Aging Process." *Journal of Gerontology* 45, No. 4, 1990, pp. 105–110.

58. R. Pamplona, M.J. Bellmunt, M. Portero, and J. Prat. "Mechanisms of Glycation in Atherogenesis." *Medical Hypotheses* 40, 1990, pp. 174–181.

59. Ibid.

60. Nancy Appleton. *Healthy Bones*. (Garden City Park, NY: Avery Publishing Group, 1991.)

61. Annette T. Lee, and Anthony Cerami. "The Role of Glycation in Aging." *Annals of the New York Academy of Science* 663, pp. 63–70.

62. Frances Sheridan Goulart. "Are You Sugar Smart?" *American Fitness*, March–April 1991, pp. 34–38.

63. Ibid.

64. Ibid.

65. Ibid.

Kurt Greenberg. "An Update on the Yeast Connection." *Health News and Review*, Spring 1990, p. 10.

66. Frances Sheridan Goulart.

"Are You Sugar Smart?" *American Fitness*, March–April 1991, pp. 34–38.

67. Ibid.

68. Ibid.

69. Ibid.

70. Ibid.

71. Jonell Nash. "Health Contenders." *Essence* 23, January 1992, pp. 79–81.

E. Grand. "Food Allergies and Migraine." *Lancet* 8126, No. 1, 1979, pp. 955–959.

72. Larry Christensen. "The Role of Caffeine and Sugar in Depression." *The Nutrition Report* 9, No. 3, March 1991, pp. 17–24.

73. Ibid.

74. Shelton Reiser, J. Hallfrisch, M. Fields, et al. "Effects of Sugars on Indices on Glucose Tolerance in Humans." *American Journal of Clinical Nutrition* 43, 1986, pp. 151–159.

75. W. Kruis, G. Forstraier, C. Scheurlen, and F. Stellaard. "Effects of Diets Low and High in Refined Sugars on Gut Transit, Bile Acid Metabolism and Bacterial Fermentation." *Gut* 32, 1991, pp. 367–370.

76. John Yudkin. "Metabolic Changes Induced by Sugar in Relation to Coronary Heart Disease and Diabe-

tes." *Nutrition and Health* 5, No. 1–2, 1987, pp. 5–8.

77. Ibid.

Chapter 6

1. Ingvar Bjarnason, P.J. Weiss, and Timothy Peters. "The Leaky Gut of Alcoholism: Possible Route of Entry for Toxic Compounds." *Lancet* 8370, January 28, 1984, pp. 178–182.

2. George A. Ulett. "Food Allergy—Cytotoxic Testing and the Central Nervous System." *Psychiatric Journal of the University of Ottawa* 5, No. 2, June 1980, pp. 100–108.

3. Ibid.

4. C. Jean Poulos, Donald Stoddard, and Kathryn Carron. *The Relationship Between Hypoglycemia and Alcoholism.*

5. Graham A. Golditz, et al. "Alcohol Intake and Relation to Diet and Obesity in Women and Children." *American Journal of Clinical Nutrition* 54, 1991, pp. 49–55.

6. P.R. MacGregor. "Alcohol and Immune Function." *Journal of the American Medical Association* 256, September 19, 1986, pp. 1474–1479.

7. DeWayne Ashmead. *Chelated Mineral Nutrition.* (Huntington Beach, CA: Institute Publishers, 1981, p. 86.)

8. J. Persson. "Alcohol and the Small Intestine." *Scandinavian Journal of Gastroenterology* 26, 1991, pp. 3–15.

9. Ruth Adams, and Frank Murray. *Megavitamin Therapy.* (New York: Larchmont Books, 1973.)

10. Sanford Bolton, Martin Feldman, and Gary Null. "A Pilot Study of Some Physiological and Psychological Effects of Caffeine." *The Journal of Orthomolecular Psychiatry* 13, No. 1, first quarter 1984, pp. 1–7.

11. D. Kerr, R.S. Sherwin, F. Pavalkin, et al. "Effects of Caffeine on the Recognition of and Responses to Hypoglycemia in Humans." *Annals of Internal Medicine* 119, 1993, pp. 799–804.

12. Sanford Bolton, and Gary Null. "Caffeine's Psychological Effects, Use and Abuse." *Journal of Orthomolecular Psychiatry* 10, No. 3, third quarter 1991, pp. 202–211.

13. Jeffrey Bland. *Your Health Under Siege.* (Brattleboro, VT: The Stephen Green Press, 1981.)

14. James F. Scheer. "Coffee: The Iron Thief." *Health Freedom News,* October 1990, p. 9.

15. Sanford Bolton, and Gary Null. "Caffeine's Psycho-

logical Effects, Use and Abuse." *Journal of Orthomolecular Psychiatry* 10, No. 3, third quarter 1991, pp. 202–211.

16. Herta Spencer, and Lois Kramer. "Antacids-Induced Calcium Loss." *Archives of Internal Medicine* 143, No. 4, 1983, pp. 657–658.

17. Ibid.

18. *The Signet/Mosby Medical Encyclopedia.* (New York: The C.V. Mosby Company, 1987.)

19. Harold E. Buttram. "Overuse of Antibiotics and the Need for Alternatives." *Townsend Letter for Doctors,* November 1991, pp. 867–869.

20. William Bennett. Oregon Health Science University, Portland, OR. Personal interview, June 10, 1986.

21. Edith Stanley, et al. "Increased Virus Shedding with Aspirin Treatment of Rhinovirus Infection." *Journal of the American Medical Association,* 231, No. 12, March 24, 1975, pp. 1248–1251.

22. Arthur Vander, James Sherman, and Dorothy Luciano. *Human Physiology.* (New York: McGraw-Hill Publishing, 1980.)

23. Edith Stanley, et al. "Increased Virus Shedding with Aspirin Treatment of Rhinovirus Infection." *Journal of*

the American Medical Association, 231, No. 12, March 24, 1975, pp. 1248–1251.

24. N.M.H. Graham. "Adverse Effects of Aspirin, Acetaminophen and Ibuprofen on Immune Function, Viral Shedding and Clinical Status in Rhinovirus-Infected Volunteers." *Journal of Infectious Diseases* 162, 1990, pp. 1277–1282.

25. Richard S. Muther, Donald M. Potter, and William Bennett. "Aspirin-Induced Depression of Glomerular Filtration Rate in Normal Humans: Role of Sodium Balance." *Annals of Internal Medicine* 94, 1981, pp. 317–321.

26. P.J. Roderick, et al. "The Gastrointestinal Toxicity of Aspirin: An Overview of Randomized Controlled Trials." *British Journal of Clinical Pharmacology* 35, 1993, pp. 219–226.

27. *Senior Counselor* (Special 1991 edition.)

28. Marlene Cimons. "New Study Strongly Links Aspirin, Reyes Syndrome." *Los Angeles Times,* February 1, 1985.

29. L. Gail Darlington. "Dietary Therapy for Arthritis." *Nutrition and Rheumatic Diseases/Rheumatic Disease Clinics*

of North America 17, No. 2, 1991, pp. 273–285.

30. C. Joas, H. Kewitz, and D. Reenhold-Kouniati. "Effects of Diuretics of Plasma Lipoproteins in Healthy Men." *European Journal of Clinical Pharmacology* 17, 1980, pp. 251–257.

31. Philip Sambrook, et al. "Prevention of Corticosteroid Osteoporosis: A Comparison of Calcium, Calcitriol, and Calcitonin." *New England Journal of Medicine* 328, No. 24, June 17, 1993, pp. 1747–1752.

32. David A. Eschenback and Philip B. Mead. "Managing Problem Vaginitis." *Patient Care*, September 15, 1992, pp. 137–152.

33. Elna Widell. "Those Allergenic Sweet Nothings in Your Pharmaceutical Pill." *Environmental Illness Association Newsletter*, July 1984.

34. W. Lyinsky, and P. Shuber. "Benzo-Pyrene and Other Polynuclear Hydrocarbons in Charbroiled Meat." *Science* 145, 1985, p. 2.

35. Leonard Bjeldanes. "Effects of High Temperatures on Meats." *Food and Chemical Toxicology* 23, No. 12, April 1985.

36. Francis M. Pottenger, Jr., and D.G. Simonsen. "Influence of Heat Labile Factors on Nutri-

tion in Oral Development and Health." *Journal of Southern California State Dental Association*, November 1939.

37. Francis M. Pottenger, Jr. *Pottengers Cats*. (La Mesa, CA: Price-Pottenger Nutrition Foundation, 1983.)

38. Mary Kerney Levenstein. *Everyday Cancer Risks and How to Avoid Them*. (Garden City Park, NY: Avery Publishing Group, 1992.)

39. M.R. Smith. "The Role of Food Additives in Intolerance Reactions to Food." *Bibliotheca Nutritio et Dieta, Nutritional Aspects and Development* 48, 1991, pp. 72–80.

40. Jack L. Samuels. "FDA's New Food Labels Ignore MSG Sensitivities." *Nutrition Week* 23, No. 10, March 12, 1993, pp. 4–5.

41. Lewis W. Mayron, and Erwin Kaplan. "The Use of Chromium-51 Sodium Chromate for the Detection of Food and Chemical Sensitivities." *Annals of Allergy* 38, 1977, p. 323.

42. Cyril Abrahams, Koshilya Rijhsinghani, and Martin Swerdlow. "Tumor Induction in Mice Following Administration of DEA-HCI and $NaNO_2$." *Cancer Detection and Prevention* 5, No.3, 1982, pp. 283–290.

43. L. Tollefson, and R.J. Barnard. "An Analysis of FDA Passive Surveillance Reports of Seizures Associated with Consumption of Aspartame." *Journal of the American Dietetic Association* 92, No.5, May 1992, pp. 598–601.

44. David Voreacos. "Experts Tell Panel of Continued Concern Over Use of Aspartame." *Los Angeles Times*, November 4, 1987, p. 19.

45. A. Kulczychi, Jr. "Aspartame-Induced Hives." *Journal of Allergy and Clinical Immunology* 2, February 1995, pp. 639–640.

   R.H. Moser. "Aspartame and Memory Loss." *Journal of the American Medical Association* 272, No. 19, November 19, 1994, p. 1543.

   J.A. Krohn. "Aspartame and Attention Deficit Disorder." *Pediatrics*, October 1994, p. 576.

   B.A. Shaywitz, and E.J. Novotny. "Aspartame and Seizures." *Neurology* 143, March 1993, pp. 630–631.

46. R.G. Walton, R. Hudak, and R.J. Green-Waite. "Adverse Reactions to Aspartame: Double-Blind Challenge in Patients from a Vulnerable Population." *Biological Psychiatry* 34, No. 1–2, July 1–15, 1993, pp. 13–17.

47. Sandra Woodruff. *Diabetic Dream Desserts*. (Garden City Park, NY: Avery Publishing Group, 1996.)

Chapter 7

1. Hans Selye. *Stress Without Distress*. (New York: Signet, 1974.)

2. *Psychosomatic Medicine* 49, September–October 1987, pp. 435, 450.

3. "Depression, Stress and Immunity." *Lancet* 8548, No. 1, June 27, 1987, pp. 1467–1468.

4. Steven Schleifer. "Clinical Consequences of Stress: The Immune Connection." (Secaucus, NJ: Network for Continuing Medical Education, 1987. Videocassette.)

5. I.I. Brekhman, and I.F. Nesterenko. *Brown Sugar and Health*. (New York: Pergamon Press, 1983.)

Chapter 8

1. Walter H. Glinsmann, Hiltje Irausquin, and Youngmee K. Park. *Report from FDA's Sugar Task Force, 1986: Evaluation of Health Aspects of Sugars Contained in Carbohydrate Sweeteners*. (Washington, DC: Center for Food Safety and Applied Nutrition, 1986, p. 39.)

2. N.W. Jerome. "Taste Experi-

ence and the Development of a Dietary Preference for Sweet in Humans." *Taste and Development: The Genesis of Sweet Preference.* Fogarty International Center Proceedings, No. 32, ed. J.M. Weiffenbach. Bethesda, MD: U.S. Department of Health, Education, and Welfare, 1977.

3. "Depression and Stress Immunity." *Lancet* 8548, No. 1, June 27, 1987, pp. 1467–1468.

4. D. Behar, J. Rapoport, Berg C. Adams, and M. Cornblat. "Sugar Challenge Testing with Children Considered Behaviorally Sugar Reactive." *Nutritional Behavior* 1, 1984, pp. 277–288.

5. Marcel Kinsbourne. "Sugar and the Hyperactive Child." *New England Journal of Medicine* 330, No. 5, February 3, 1994, p. 355.

6. J. Goldman, et al. "Behavioral

Effects of Sucrose on Preschool Children." *Journal of Abnormal Psychology* 14, 1986, pp. 565–577.

7. Alex Schauss. *Diet, Crime, and Delinquency.* (Berkeley, CA: Parker House, 1981.)

8. Anne Schick. "Fast Food, Couch Potato Lifestyle Taking Toll on Youth." *Family Practice News,* April 1, 1992, p. 28.

9 R. Troncone, et al. "Increased Intestinal Sugar Permeability After Challenge in Children with Cow's Milk Allergy or Intolerance." *Allergy* 49, 1994, pp. 142–146.

Chapter 9

1. Mary Kerney Levenstein. *Everyday Cancer Risks and How to Avoid Them.* (Garden City Park, NY: Avery Publishing Group, 1992.)

2. Ibid.

Selected
Bibliography

Abrahams, Cyril, Koshilya Rijhsinghani, and Martin Swerdlow. "Tumor Induction in Mice Following Administration of DEA-HCl and NaNO2." *Cancer Detection and Prevention* 5, No. 3, 1982.

Abrahamson, E.M., and A.W. Pezet. *Body, Mind and Sugar.* New York: Avon Books, 1951.

Adams, Ruth, and Frank Murray. *Megavitamin Therapy.* New York: Larchmont Books, 1973.

Appleton, Nancy. *Healthy Bones.* Garden City Park, NY: Avery Publishing Group, 1989.

Ashmead, DeWayne. *Chelated Mineral Nutrition.* Huntington Beach, CA: Institute Publishers, 1981.

Balch, James F., and Phyllis A. Balch. *Prescription for Nutritional Healing.* Garden City Park, NY: Avery Publishing Group, 1996.

Bjarnason, Ingvar, Kevin Ward, and Timothy Peters. "The Leaky Gut of Alcoholism: Possible Route of Entry for Toxic Compounds." *Lancet* 8370, January 28, 1984.

Bjeldanes, Leonard. "Effects of High Temperatures on Meat." *Journal of Food and Chemical Toxicology* 23, No. 12, April 1985.

Bland, Jeffrey. *Digestive Enzymes*. New Canaan, CT: Keats Publishing, 1983.

———. *Your Health Under Siege*. Brattleboro, VT: The Stephen Green Press, 1981.

Braganza, J.M. "Selenium Deficiency, Cystic Fibrosis, and Pancreatic Cancer." *Lancet* 2: 1238, 1986.

Brekhman, I.I., and I.F. Nesterenko. *Brown Sugar and Health*. New York: Pergamon Press, 1983.

Brown, H. Harrow. "The Diagnosis and Management of Allergy." Paper delivered at the annual meeting of the Indian College of Allergy and Immunology, Simla, AZ, September 1980.

Buckley, Rebecca. "Food Allergy." *Journal of the American Medical Association* 248: 26–27, 1982.

Cannon, G. "The Sugar Lobby." *Lancet*, January 26, 1985.

Canon, Walter B. *The Wisdom of the Body*, 2nd ed. New York: Norton and Company, 1963.

Carroll, Lewis. *Alice's Adventures in Wonderland*. New York: Bantam Books, 1981.

Catterall, William E. "Rheumatoid Arthritis Is an Allergy." *Arthritis News Today*, 1980.

Challem, Jack Joseph, and Renate Lewin. "Vitamins and Fiber for Preventing Gallstones." *Let's Live*, April 14, 1984, pp. 10–12.

Cheraskin, E., and W.M. Ringsdorf, Jr., with Arline Brecher. *Psychodietetics*. New York: Bantam Books, 1978.

Cimons, Marlene. "New Study Strongly Links Aspirin, Reye's Syndrome." *Los Angeles Times*, February 1, 1985.

Cleave, T.L. *The Saccharine Disease*. New Canaan, CT: Keats Publishing, 1974.

Cleave, T.L., and G.D. Campbell. *Diabetes, Coronary Thrombosis, and the Saccharine Disease*. Bristol, England: John Wright & Sons, 1969.

Coca, Arthur F. *The Pulse Test.* New York: Arco Publishing Company, 1978.

Cohn, Mark Nathan. *The Rise of Civilization.* New Haven, CT: Yale University Press, 1989.

Crook, William G. *The Yeast Connection.* Jackson, TN: Professional Books, 1984.

Darlington, L.G., N.W. Ramsey, and J.R. Mansfield. "Placebo-Controlled, Blind Study of Dietary Manipulation Therapy in Rheumatoid Arthritis." *Lancet,* February 6, 1986, pp. 36–38.

Davenport, H.W. "Why the Stomach Does Not Digest Itself." *Scientific American* 226: 87–93, January 1972.

Deerr, N. *The History of Sugar.* London: Chapman & Hall Co., 1949.

Doisy, R.J. *Minerals and Trace Elements.* pp. 586–594. (Publisher unknown.)

Douglass, John M. "Psoriasis and Diet." *Western Journal of Medicine* 133: 450, November 1980.

Dufty, William. *Sugar Blues.* New York: Warner Books, 1975.

Egger, J., et al. "Is Migraine Food Allergy?" *Lancet,* October 15, 1983, pp. 865–867.

Erlander, Stig R. "The Cause and Cure of Multiple Sclerosis." *The Diet to End Disease* 1: 59–63, No. 3, March 3, 1979.

Frame, Boy, and Geoffrey Marel. "Reflections on Bone Disease in Total Parenteral Nutrition." In *Metabolic Bone Disease in Total Parenteral Nutrition.* Jack W. Coburn, and Gordon L. Klein, eds. Baltimore: Urban and Schwarzenberg, 1985.

Gaby, Alan R. *The Doctor's Guide to Vitamin B_6.* Emmaus, PA: Rodale Press, 1983.

Galton, Lawrence. *You May Not Need a Psychiatrist.* New York: Simon & Schuster, 1979.

Garmon, Linda. "Crohn's Disease: Intestinal Enigma." *Science News* 177: 280–281, May 3, 1980.

Gerstenzang, Sharon D. *Cook With Me Sugar Free*. New York: Simon & Schuster, 1983.

Glinsmann, Walter H., Hiltje Irausquin, and Youngmee K. Park. *Report from FDA's Sugar Task Force, 1986: Evaluation of Health Aspects of Sugars Contained in Carbohydrate Sweeteners*. Washington, DC: Center for Food Safety and Applied Nutrition, 1986.

Goldburg Group, Burton. *Alternative Medicine*. Payallup, WA: Future Medicine Publishing, Inc. 1993.

Goulart, Frances Sheridan. "Behind Bars, Kicking the Candy Bar Habit." *Herbalist New Health*, January and February 1981.

Grant, Ellen. "Food Allergy and Migraine." *Lancet* 8123: 966–969, 1979.

Hallfrisch, J., et al. "The Effects of Fructose on Blood Lipid Levels." *American Journal of Clinical Nutrition* 37:740–748, No. 5, 1983.

Heaton, K.W. "The Sweet Road to Gallstones." *British Medical Journal* 288:1103–1104, April 14, 1984.

Hill, Amelia Nathan. Amelia Nathan Hill International Foundation of Collating Allergy Research, Wimbledon, England, April 3, 1983. Personal interview.

Historical Statistics of the U.S.—Colonial Times to 1970. Washington, DC: U.S. Government Printing Office, 1975, p. 65.

Hunter, Beatrice Trum. *Food Additives and Your Health*. New Canaan, CT: Keats Publishing, 1972.

———. *The Sugar Primer*. Charlotte, NC: Garden Way Publishing, 1979.

———. *The Sugar Trap and How to Avoid It*. Boston: Houghton Mifflin Co., 1982.

Jenkins, David, et al. "Glycemic Index of Foods: A Physiological Basis for Carbohydrate Exchange." *American Journal of Clinical Nutrition* 34: 360–366.

Joas, C., H. Kewitz, and D. Reenhold-Kouniati. "Effects of Diuretics of Plasma Lipoproteins in Healthy Men." *European Journal of Clinical Pharmacology* 17: 251–257, 1980.

Jones, V.A., et al. "Crohn's Disease: Maintenance of Remission by Diet." *Lancet*, July 27, 1985, pp. 177–180.

Jones, V.A., et al. "Food Intolerance: A Major Factor in the Pathogenesis of Irritable Bowel Syndrome." *Lancet*, November 10, 1982, pp. 1115–1117.

Kaslow, Arthur L., and Richard B. Miles. *Freedom From Chronic Disease*. Los Angeles: J.P. Tarcher, 1979.

Keen, H., B. Thomas, R. Jarrett, and L. Fuller. "Nutritional Intake, Adiposity, and Diabetes." *British Medical Journal* 1: 655–658, 1989.

Kelsey, J., et al., "Diets High in Fructose or Sucrose in Young Women." *American Journal of Clinical Nutrition* 27: 926–936, 1994.

Kijak, Ernest, George Foust, and Ralph Steinman. "Relationship of Blood Sugar Level and Leukocytic Phagocytosis." *Southern California State Dental Association Journal* 32, No. 9, September 1964.

King, Glen W. *Statistical Abstracts of the U.S., 1993*. Washington, DC: U.S. Government Printing Office, 1993.

Klenner, Frederick Robert. "Significance of High Daily Intake of Ascorbic Acid in Preventive Medicine." In *A Physician's Handbook to Orthomolecular Medicine*. Roger Williams, and Dwight K. Kalita, eds. New York: Pergamon Press, 1978.

Kozlovsky, A., et al. "Effects of Diets High in Simple Sugars on Urinary Chromium Losses," *Metabolism* 35: 515–518, June 1986.

Kupsinel, Roy. "A Patient's Guide to Mercury Amalgam Toxicity." Oviedo, FL: Keeps Komments, 1984.

Lazarus, Pat. "Multiple Sclerosis and Amyotrophic Lateral Sclerosis: More Hope Than We Think." *Let's Live*, April 1980, pp. 70–77.

LeShan, Lawrence. *You Can Fight for Your Life*. New York: Evans Publishing Co., 1980.

Levenstein, Mary Kerney. *Everyday Cancer Risks and How to Avoid Them*. Garden City Park, NY: Avery Publishing Group, 1992.

Levine, Stephen. "Oxidants and Antioxidants and Chemical Sensitivities." *Allergy Research Review* 2, No. 1, Spring 1981.

Linn, Margaret, et al. Cited in *American Institute for Cancer Research Information Sheet*, 1985.

Liversidge, L.A. "Treatment and Management of Multiple Sclerosis." *British Medical Bulletin* 33:78–83, 1977.

Lorenzani, Shirley. "Candida Albicans." Cassette tapes, sets I and II. La Mesa, CA: Price-Pottenger Nutrition Foundation, 1978.

Lyinsky, W., and P. Shuber. "Benzo-Pyrene and Other Polynuclear Hydrocarbons in Charbroiled Meat." *Science* 145: 2, 1985.

Mayron, Lewis W., and Erwin Kaplan. "The Use of Chromium—51 Sodium Chromate for the Detection of Food and Chemical Sensitivities." *Annals of Allergy* 38: 323, 1977.

McKenzie, M.M. "Urinary Excretion of Cadmium, Zinc and Copper in Normotensive and Hypertensive Women." *New England Medical Journal* 80: 68–70.

Moerman, Clara J., et al. "Dietary Sugar Intake in the Etiology of Biliary Tract Cancer." *Internal Journal of Epidemiology* 22: 207–214, 1990.

Mohammed, Abdel Rahim, et al. "Osteoporosis and Periodontal Disease: A review." *California Dental Association Journal*, March 1994, pp. 69–74.

Morris, Brian W., et al. "Trace Element Chromium—A Role in Glucose Homeostasis," *American Journal of Clinical Nutrition* 55: 989–991, 1992.

Muther, Richard S., Donald M. Potter, and William Bennett. "Aspirin-Induced Depression of Glomerular Filtration Rate in Normal Humans: Role of Sodium Balance." *Annals of Internal Medicine* 94: 317–321, 1981.

Notelovitz, Morris, and Marsha Ware. *Stand Tall: Every Woman's Guide to Preventing Osteoporosis*. New York: Bantam Books, 1985.

Null, Gary. "A Trio of Distinguished Doctors Discuss Successful MS Treatment." *Bestways*, October 1981, pp. 35–40.

"Osteoporosis in Young Men." *Healthwise* 6, No. 1, January 1983.

Pacetti, Bruce, and Nancy Appleton. *How to Monitor Your Basic Health*. Santa Monica, CA: Choice Publishing Co., 1985.

Page, Melvin. *Body Chemistry in Health and Disease*. La Mesa, CA: Price-Pottenger Nutrition Foundation.

Page, Melvin, and H. Leon Abram, Jr. *Your Body Is Your Best Doctor*. New Canaan, CT: Keats Publishing, 1972.

Pariza, Michael W., *Diet and Cancer*. Summit, NJ: American Council on Science and Health, 1985.

Pearson, D.J., K. Rix, and S. Bently. "Food Allergy, How Much in the Mind." *Lancet* 2:1259–1261, 1983.

Petitpierre, M., P. Guimowski, and J.P. Girard. "Irritable Bowel Syndrome and Hypersensitivity to Food." *Annals of Allergy* 54: 538–540, June 1985.

Philpott, William H., and Dwight K. Kalita. *Brain Allergies*. New Canaan, CT: Keats Publishing, 1980.

Philpott, William H., and Dwight K. Kalita. *Victory Over Diabetes*. New Canaan, CT: Keats Publishing, 1983.

Pottenger, Francis M., Jr. *Pottenger's Cats*. La Mesa, CA: Price-Pottenger Nutrition Foundation, 1983.

Poulos, Jean. "The Nutritional Approach to Osteoporosis." *Nutritional Consultant*, February 1984, p. 25.

Power, Lawrence. "Change in Diet May Help Relieve Asthma Patient." *Los Angeles Times*, May 7, 1985.

Power, Lawrence. "Sensitivity: You React to What You Eat." *Los Angeles Times*, February 12, 1985.

Power, Lawrence. "Special Diets Ease Some Headache Pain." *Los Angeles Times*, August 12, 1984.

Prescott, L.F. "Analgesic Nephropathy." *Drugs* 23: 75–149, 1982.

Raboff, J. "Oxidized Lipids: A Key to Heart Disease." *Science News* 129: 278.

Randolph, Theron G. "Is Allergy the Root of Alcoholism?" *Bestways*, March 1983, pp. 44–49.

Randolph, Theron G., and Ralph W. Moss. *An Alternative Approach to Allergies.* New York: Bantam Books, 1981.

Randolph, Theron G., and Leona B. Yeager. "Corn Sugar as an Allergen." *Annals of Allergy,* September–October 1949, pp. 650–661.

Rea, William, et al. "Food and Chemical Susceptibility After Environmental Chemical Overexposure: Case Histories." *Annals of Allergy* 41: 101–110, August 1978.

Reiser, S. "Effects of Dietary Sugars on Metabolic Risk Factors Associated with Heart Disease." *Nutritional Health* 3, 1985.

Ringsdorf, W., E. Cheraskin, and E. Ramsey. "Sucrose Neutrophilic Phagocytosis and Resistance to Disease." *Dental Survey* 52, No. 12, 1976.

Ritter, E.J., et al. "Potentiative Interaction Between Caffeine and Various Teratogenic Agents." *Teratology* 25, No. 95, 1982.

Roberts, H.J. *Aspartame—Nutrasweet: Is It Safe?* Philadelphia, PA: Charles Press Publishers, 1984.

———. "Reactions Attributed to Aspartame—Containing Products: 551 Cases." *Journal of Applied Nutrition* 40:85–94, 1988.

Robinson, Miles H. "On Sugar and White Flour—the Dangerous Twins." In *A Physician's Handbook to Orthomolecular Medicine.* Roger Williams, and Dwight K. Kalita, eds. New York: Pergamon Press, 1978.

Rogers, S. "Sugar and Health." *Lancet,* February 23, 1985.

Rose Elizabeth. *Lady of Gray.* Santa Monica, CA: Butterfly Publishing Co., 1985.

Sanchez, A. et al. "Role of Sugars in Human Neutrophilic Phagocytosis." *American Journal of Clinical Nutrition,* November 1973, pp. 1180–1184.

Saner, G. "Urinary Chromium Excretion During Pregnancy and Relationship With Intravenous Glucose Loading." *American Journal of Clinical Nutrition* 34:1676, 1981.

Schauss, Alexander. *Diet, Crime, and Delinquency.* Berkeley, CA: Parker House, 1981.

Schleifer, Steven, et al. "A Simplified Method for Assaying PHA Induced Stimulation of Rat Peripheral Blood Lymphocytes." *Journal of Immunological Methods* 51:287–291, No. 3, 1982.

Schneider, Keith. "'Miracle Cure'—Holism or Hokum?" *New Age*, September 1985, p. 12.

Selye, Hans. *The Stress of Life*. San Francisco: McGraw-Hill, 1978.

———. *Stress Without Distress*. New York: Signet, 1974.

Shames, Richard L. "About AIDS." *Holistic Health*, November 1985, pp. 26–28.

Shannon, Ira L. *Brand Name Guide to Sugar*. Chicago: Nelson Hall, 1977.

Shurkin, Joel N. "Artificial Sweeteners." *Healthline*, October 1983, p. 10.

"Sugar Substitutes." *Medical Hotline* 4: 1, No. 4, April–May 1983.

Smith, Lendon H. *Feed Yourself Right*. New York: Dell Publishing Co., 1983.

———. *Improving Your Child's Behavior Chemistry*. New York: Pocket Books, 1976.

Spencer, Herta, and Lois Kramer. "Antacids-Induced Calcium Loss." *Archives of Internal Medicine* 143: 657–658, No. 4, 1983.

Stanley, Edith, et al. "Increased Virus Shedding With Aspirin Treatment of Rhinovirus Infection." *Journal of the American Medical Association*, March 24, 1975.

Stead, R.J., et al. "Selenium Deficiency and Possible Increased Risk of Carcinoma in Adults With Cystic Fibrosis." *Lancet* 2: 862, 1986.

Tauroso, Nicola Michael. "Allergy and Sensitivities." *Living Health Bulletin* 2:13–14, 1984.

Truss, C. Orion. *The Missing Diagnosis*. Birmingham, AL: C. Truss, 1983.

———. "Restoration of Immunologic Competence to Candida Albicans." *Orthomolecular Psychiatry* 9: 287–301, No. 4, 1980.

Ulett, George A. "Food Allergy—Cytotoxic Testing and the Central Nervous System." *Psychiatric Journal of the University of Ottawa* 5: 100–108, No. 2, June 1980.

United States Sugar Policy: An Analysis. Washington, D.C.: U.S. Government Printing Office, 1989.

Vander, Arthur, James Sherman, and Dorothy Luciano. *Human Physiology.* New York: McGraw-Hill Publishing, 1980.

Wade, Carlson. *Helping Your Health With Enzymes.* New York: ARC Books, 1971.

Wallach, Joel. "Metabolic Therapy for Heart Disease, Cancer, Allergies, and Multiple Sclerosis." Paper presented at the National Health Federation, Long Beach, CA, January 1983. Tape.

Wallach, J.D., and B. Germaise. "Cystic Fibrosis: A Perinatal Manifestation of Selenium Deficiency." *Trace Substances in Environmental Health.* D.D. Hemphill, ed. Columbia, MO: University of Missouri Press, 1979.

Wallis, Claudia. "Stress—Can We Cope?" *Time,* June 6, 1983, pp. 48–54.

Warberg, Otto. *The Metabolism of Tumours.* London: Constable & Co., 1930.

Widell, Elna. "Those Allergenic Sweet Nothings in Your Pharmaceutical Pill." *Environmental Illness Association Newsletter,* July 1984.

Wiggins, Roger C., and M.P. Cochrane. "Immune Complex—Medicated Biological Effects." *New England Journal of Medicine* 304: 518, 1981.

Willeke, K., and K. Whitley. "Aerosols: Size Distribution Interpretation." *Air Pollution Control Association Journal* 25: 196, No. 526.

Wilson, David A. *What You Should Know About Sugar and Food Additives.* Black Mountain, NC: Loren House, 1975.

Wilson, Eva D., Katherine H. Fisher, and Pilar A. Garcia. *Principles of Nutrition.* New York: John Wiley & Sons, 1979.

Wolf, R.N., and S.M. Grundy. "Influence of Exchanging Carbohydrate for Saturated Fatty Acids on Plasma Lipids and Lipoproteins in Men." *Journal of Nutrition* 113: 1521, 1983.

Woodruff, Sandra. *Diabetic Dream Desserts*. Garden City Park, NY: Avery Publishing Group, 1996.

Yudkin, John. "Dietary Fat and Dietary Sugar in Relation to Ischemic Heart Disease and Diabetes." *Lancet* 2, No. 4, 1964.

———. "Sugar and Disease." *Nature* 239: 197–199.

———. "Sugar for Debate." *Lancet*, March 30, 1985.

Yudkin, J., S. Kang, and K. Bruckdorf. "Effects of High Dietary Sugar." *British Journal of Medicine*, November 22, 1980, p. 1396.

Ziff, Sam. *The Toxic Time Bomb*. New York: Aurora Press, 1984.

Zack, Maura, and Wilbur D. Currier. *Sugar Isn't Always Sweet*. Brea, CA: Uplift Books, 1983.

Zucker, Martin. "Fight Back! Don't Learn to Live With M.S." *Let's Live*, December 1982, pp. 10–14.

———. "Nutrition and the Addicted." *Let's Live*, June 1980, p. 16.

AUDIO CASSETTES

The following audio cassette tapes present information on a variety of subjects. An order form is provided on the following page.

Lick the Sugar Habit—An introduction to the book, this tape provides detailed explanations of the body chemistry principle, mineral relationships, the endocrine system, enzymes, and promoters of infectious and degenerative diseases. (1 hour)

Allergies—What are food allergies? What causes them? How can they be eliminated? Learn how foods to which you have an allergic reaction can be reintroduced in your diet. Environmental allergies are also discussed. (1 hour)

Osteoporosis—Although you may be getting a reasonable amount of calcium in your diet, if your body chemistry is upset, the calcium cannot be absorbed properly. This tape explains how to look for symptoms of calcium deficiency and how to test for susceptibility to osteoporosis. (1 hour)

Obesity—The latest research on the relationship of allergies, addictions, and cravings to obesity is presented. (30 minutes) **Women** is on flip side of tape.

Women—Information on premenstrual syndrome (PMS), candidiasis (yeast infections), menstruation, menopause, and postmenopausal problems is provided. (30 minutes) **Obesity** is on flip side of tape.

Children—This tape begins with a discussion of prenatal nutrition. Information on food allergies and eating problems for infants and children follows. Ideas for encouraging older children and teenagers to eat nutritious foods end the tape. (1 hour)

Food Preparation—This tape answers the following questions: Where can I shop for the best, most nutritious foods? How can I best prepare food to keep it from upsetting the body's chemical balance? What should I know about food additives, irradiation, insecticides, and fungicides? (1 hour)

Urine and pH Testing—Information and instructions for testing homeostasis through saliva and urine are presented. Common causes of upset body chemistry are discussed, as well as ways to regain the body's chemical balance. (1 hour)

AUDIO CASSETTE
Order Form

Name: _____

Address: _____ Apt.:_____

City:_____

State: _____ Zip: _____

List Cassette Titles:

1. _____ 5._____

2. _____ 6. _____

3. _____ 7._____

4. _____ 8. _____

* Price List:

Quantity	Price	Shipping	Shipping to Canada (U.S. currency)
1	$ 6.00	$ 1.25	$ 1.50
2	12.00	1.50	1.75
3	15.00	1.75	2.00
4	20.00	2.00	2.25
5	25.00	2.25	2.50
6	30.00	2.50	2.75
7	35.00	2.75	3.00
8	40.00	3.00	3.25

* **California Residents Only**, please apply appropriate sales tax or 10%.

Mail this completed form, along with a check made payable to Nancy Appleton, Ph.D., to:

Nancy Appleton, Ph.D.
PO Box 3083
Santa Monica, CA 90403

BODY CHEMISTRY TEST KIT
Order Form

This kit includes tests that determine if your body chemistry is balanced. Solution for 250 tests, two test tubes, an eye dropper, a brush for cleaning the test tubes, and pH paper to test the acidity-alkalinity of saliva is included. An informative booklet, *Monitoring Your Basic Health*, which contains information on body chemistry— what upsets it and how to regain and maintain its balance—is also included. This booklet also offers suggested food plans and instructions on how to test for food allergies.

Name: _____

Address: _____ Apt.:_____

City:_____

State: _____ Zip: _____

* Cost of Body Chemistry Test Kit

1 kit	$ 20.00
Shipping	2.50
Shipping to Canada (U.S. currency)	3.00

* California Residents Only, please apply appropriate sales tax or 10%.

Mail this completed form, along with a check made payable to Nancy Appleton, Ph.D., to:

Nancy Appleton, Ph.D.
PO Box 3083
Santa Monica, CA 90403

About
the Author

Nancy Appleton earned her BS in clinical nutrition from UCLA and her PhD in health services from Walden University. She maintains a private practice in Los Angeles, California. An avid researcher, Dr. Appleton lectures extensively throughout the world and has appeared on numerous television and radio talk shows. In addition to *Lick the Sugar Habit*, she is also the author of the best-selling *Healthy Bones* and *Secrets of Natural Healing with Food*.

Index

Acidophilus, 101
Acidosis, 49
Acquired immune
    deficiency syndrome.
    See AIDS.
Adams, Dr. Ruth, 114
Adrenaline, 141
Advanced Glycated
    Proteins (AGEs),
    55, 56
AGEs. *See* Advanced
    Glycated Proteins.
AIDS, 160
Alcohol, 83, 111–115, 180
Alcoholism, sugar and,
    113
Allergic reaction
    acute, 45–46
    chronic, 46–49

degenerative,
    49–51
Allergies, environmental,
    39–41
Allergies, food
    addiction and, 47–49
    alcohol and, 112
    aspirin and, 124
    asthma and, 75
    arthritis and, 74
    chemical exposure
        and, 40
    development of, 31,
        35–36, 43, 44, 74
    digestion and, 33, 37,
        38, 42, 49
    headaches and, 76
    in infants, 36, 37
    infections and, 38

multiple sclerosis and,
    100
self-test for, 6
stages of, 45–51
sugar's role in, 34, 35,
    39, 92
symptoms of, 33
Aluminum, 83, 119
Alzheimer's disease, 83
Amadori products, 56
American Chemical
    Society, 88
Analgesics, 124
Anorexia nervosa, 94
Antacids, 119–120
Antibiotics, 121
Arthritis, 73–74
Arthritis News Today, 74
Artificial sweeteners,
    131–133, 178
Ashmead, Dr. DeWayne,
    135
Aspartame, 131–133
Aspirin, 122–124
Asthma, 75–76

Basic Mayonnaise, 194
Basic Pie Crust, 197
Beet sugar, 57
Benzo(a)pyrene, 126
Berkeley Wellness Letter
    (University of
    California), 16
Biological Stress

Syndrome. *See*
    General Adaptation
    Syndrome.
Bland, Dr. Jeffrey, 117
Blood clotting, 57
Blood glucose. *See* Blood
    sugar.
Blood sugar
    carbohydrates and,
        175–176
    caffeine and, 116
    diabetes and, 64
    protein and, 177
    stress and, 141, 142
    sugar and, 13, 55, 56,
        60, 61, 90, 92, 113,
        173–174, 180
    See also Diabetes;
        Glucose; Hyper-
        glycemia; Hypo-
        glycemia.
Body Chemistry
    Principle, xi
Body Chemistry Test, 34,
    67, 73, 77, 85, 161,
    243
Breakfast, food sugges-
    tions for, 170
Brekhman, Dr. I.I.,
    141–142
British Medical Journal,
    103
*Broccoli and Potatoes
    Vinaigrette*, 196

Broccoli Soup with Vegetables, 186
Browning reaction. *See* Maillard Reaction.
Bulgarian Bean Salad, 194

Cabbage Scramble, 188
Caffeine, 76, 82, 115–118
Calcium
  candidiasis and, 95
  drugs and, 119
  function of, 21
  homeostasis and, 161–162
  mineral relationships and, 25–27
  osteoporosis and, 80–86
  sugar and, 22, 23, 89–90
  tooth decay and, 98
  See also Calcium-phosphorus ratio; Minerals; Phosphorus.
Calcium-phosphorus ratio, 25–27, 89–90, 138, 161–162
  sugar's effect on the, 22, 23, 30, 34, 63, 81, 82, 98
Calories, 91, 92, 93
Cancer, 78–80
Candida Albicans Yeast-Free Cookbook (Connolly), 193
Candidiasis, 95–97, 121, 125, 146
Cane sugar, 57
Canker sores, 102
Carbohydrates, 175–176
Carob Mousse, 197
Catecholamines, 116
Catterall, Dr. William, 74
CDC. *See* Centers for Disease Control.
Centers for Disease Control (CDC), 124
Chemical balance
  body mechanics and, 158–159
  body structure and, 159–160
  eating habits and, 157
  emotion and, 155–157
  food plans and, 165–172
Children's health, sugar and, 146–152
Chocolate, 90–91, 178
Cholesterol, 57, 88–89, 90, 117
Chromium, 16, 64, 88, 90, 179–180
Cigarette smoking, 44, 82
Cobalt, 16
Coca, Dr. Arthur F., 6

Coconut Sweet-Potato Pudding, 198
Coffee, 180
Colon cleansing, 67
Connolly, Pat, 193
Constipation, 65–67
Contact inhibition, 79
Cook, Dr. James D., 117–118
Copper, 16, 90
Corn products, 175
Corn sugar, 57
Corn syrup, 9, 10. *See also* High fructose corn syrup.
Cornstarch, 125
Corticosteroids, 125
Crohn's disease. *See* Inflammatory bowel disease.
Crook, Dr. William, 146
Curried Peppers and Garbanzos, 188
Cystic fibrosis, 104–105

"Degenerative disease process," 11–12, 19, 24, 49–51, 105
Dessert recipes, 197–199
Dextrine, 9, 57
Dextrose, 9, 10, 57, 146
Diabetes, 52, 62–65, 112, 141
"Dietary Goals for the United States" (U.S. Senate Select Committee on Dietary Goals for the United States), 14
Diuretics, 125
Douglass, Dr. John M., 77
Drugs, 118–125
Dunaif, George, 127

Eating Habits, health-promoting, 171–172
Electromagnetic fields, 158–159
Endocrine system, 70
    distress and the, 141
    genetic blueprint of the, 105–108
    sugar's effect on the, 27–30, 38–39, 60, 62, 65
Entreé recipes, 192–193
Environmental allergies. *See* Allergies, environmental.
Enzymes
    cancer and, 78
    exhaustion of, 37, 38, 42, 44 49, 112
    minerals and, 31, 33, 74, 90
    role of, 30, 126
    sugar's effect on, 34, 35, 55, 82

Equal sugar substitute, 131
"Estimated Annual Production and Consumption of Soft Drinks" (Soft Drink Association), 15–16
Estrogen therapy, 86–87
Exercise, 86, 149, 178

Fasting, 52
Fats, overheated, 125–126
Fiber, 35, 65–66, 67
Food addiction, 47–49, 92
    withdrawl from, 162
Food additives, 129–131, 147
Food allergies. *See* Allergies, food.
"Food and Drug Administration 1986 Report on Sugar Consumption," 14–15
Food plans, 162–164
Free radicals, 73, 74, 78, 79, 126, 127
Fructose, 9, 13, 57, 90, 180
Fruit, 180

Gallstones, 103
Garbure Soup, 183

General Adaptation Syndrome, 43–44
Genetic blueprints, 105–107
Gingery Chicken Soup, 185
Glucose, 13, 17, 56, 90, 125, 141, 180
Glucose tolerance factor (GTF), 179–180
Glutamic acid, 179
Glycated protein, 55
Golditz, Graham, 113
Graham, Dr. N.M.H., 123
GTF. *See* Glucose tolerance factor.

Hallfrisch, Dr. J, 90
Headaches, 76–77
Health maintenance, principles for, 154–155. *See also* Chemical balance.
Heart disease, 57, 87–91, 125
Hearty Beef Borscht, 184
HFCS. *See* High fructose corn syrup.
High fructose corn syrup (HFCS), 9, 17, 57
Holistic health, definition of, 24
Homeostastis, 45, 47, 50, 79, 95, 99

being out of, 7, 23, 49,
74
definition of, 23–24
food plans for attaining, 162–172, 180
testing for, 161–162
See also Chemical balance.
Honey, 10
Hot Asparagus Soup, 184
Hot Borscht, 187
Hydrochloric acid, 72, 120, 130
Hydrogenated oil, 91
Hyperactivity, 146–147
Hyperglycemia. *See* Diabetes.
Hypoglycemia
alcohol and, 112, 113
caffeine and, 117
sugar and, 60–65, 174, 175, 179

Immune complexes, 73
Immune system
allergies and the, 45, 46, 50, 51
antibiotics and the, 121
improving the, 161–162
psychological distress and the, 139–140
sugar's effect on the, 51–52, 53, 56, 57, 95

Inflammatory bowel disease, 101–102
Insulin
artificial sweeteners and, 178
caffeine and, 116, 117
diabetes and, 63
hypoglycemia and, 60, 61, 62
sugar consumption and, 65, 141, 174
Iodine, 17
Irausquin, Dr. Hiltje, 15
Irish Stew, 193
Iron, 21, 66, 117, 118
Islets of Langerhans, 60, 63

Kaslow, Dr. Arthur, 100
Kidney stones, 103–104
Kidneys, effect of aspirin on, 123
Kummerow, Fred. A., 89

Labels, food, 176
Lactose, 125
Lentil Tomato Loaf, 191
LeShan, Dr. Lawrence, 140
Leukocytes, 122, 123
L-glutamine. *See* Glutamic acid.
Life expectancy, current U.S., 59

Lincoln, Abraham, 14
Linn, Dr. Margaret, 140
Liver cleansing, 77

Macro minerals, 25
Magnesium, 16, 21, 27,
    85, 90, 98, 125
Maillard, Louis, 54
Maillard Reaction, 54–55
Manganese, 16
*Manhattan Clam Chowder,
    Mexican Style*, 186
Maple syrup, 10
Mayron, Dr. Lewis,
    129–130
Mercury, 134–135
Metabolism, 30, 31, 65
Methanol, 132
Minerals
    depletion of, 93
    enzymes and, 31, 33,
        42, 78, 90
    functions of, 21, 104
    relationships, 25–27,
        74, 84, 87, 97, 119,
        141, 154, 160, 162
    sugar's effect on,
        22–23, 24, 88, 91, 126
    See also Calcium-phos-
        phorus ratio.
Molded Chicken Salad,
    195
Monosodium glutamate
    (MSG), 76, 129

Monte, Dr. Woodrow C.,
    132
MSG. *See* Monosodium
    glutamate.
Multiple sclerosis (MS),
    100

Nash, Ogden, 115
Nitrates, 130
NutraSweet. *See* Aspar-
    tame.

Obesity, 92
    in children, 149
Orange juice, 34–35
Osteoporosis, 80–87
Overcooked food,
    126–128

Page, Dr. Melvin,
    22–23
Pancreas, 60, 64, 116,
    174
Pepper Slaw, 196
Periodontal disease, 85
*Persian Lamb and Bean
    Stew*, 192
Phagocytic index, 51–52,
    53
Philpott, Dr. William, 64,
    88, 90
Phosphoric acid, 180
Phosphorus, 21, 84, 98,
    119, 161–162. *See also*

Calcium-phosphorus
ratio.
Platelets, 122, 123
PMS. *See* Premenstrual
syndrome.
Polyphenols. *See* Tannic
acid.
Pottenger, Dr. Francis,
106, 127
Poulos, Jean, 112
Premenstrual syndrome
(PMS), 94–95
Prostaglandins, 122
Protein,
digestion of, 37–38,
127
glycation of, 55, 56
osteoporosis and, 84
Psoriasis, 77–78
Psychological distress,
138–140
handling, 143–144
sugar and, 140–143
See also Stress.
Psychoneuroimmunol-
ogy, 138
Pulse Test (Coca), 6
Pumpkin Pie, 198
Pyorrhea. *See* Periodontal
disease.

Randolph, Dr. Theron,
35
Ratatouille, 190

Rea, Dr. William J., 40
Refined sugar
diabetes and, 64–65
foods that contain, 7–8,
17
nutritional makeup of,
11, 13, 16
types of, 7
Reye's syndrome, 124

Saccharin, 133, 178
Salad and salad-dressing
recipes, 194–196
Savory Pepper Pilaf, 190
Schauss, Dr. Alex, 147
Schiff's base, 56
Schleifer, Dr. Steven, 140
Schneeman, Barbara,
127
Select Committee on
Nutrition and
Human Needs
(United States
Senate), 14
Selye, Dr. Hans, 43, 45
Serotonin, 132
Simple sugar. *See* Refined
sugar.
Snacks, suggestions for,
170, 176
Sodium, 83
Soft Drink Association, 15
Soft drinks, 15–16, 56, 180
Soup recipes, 183–187

*Spanish-style Rice and
    Ground Beef*, 193
*Spicy Bohemian-Style
    Tomato Soup*, 187
Spicy Carob Brownies, 199
Stanley, Dr. Edith, 122,
    123
Steinman, Ralph, 99
Stoddard, Donald, 112
Stomach acid, 81
Stomach gas, 72–73
Stress, 43–44, 137–138,
    181. *See also* Psycho-
    logical distress.
Stress Without Distress
    (Selye), 43
Sucrose, 9, 17, 147
Sugar
    America's consump-
    tion of, 9–10, 11, 14,
    15, 16, 17, 21, 55,
    145
    definition of, 17
    digestion of, 16–17, 31,
    35
    foods that contain
    "hidden," 10–11, 114
    history of, 17–18, 57
    ill effects of, 68–72
    immune system and,
    51–52, 53, 56, 57
Sugar addiction
    author's experiences
    with, 3–7, 11–12

combatting, 115,
    174–182
developing, 13, 18,
    173–174
diagnosing, 8–9
manifestations of, 12,
    18, 19, 48–49
Sugar beets, 9, 17
Sugar cane, 9, 17
*Sugar and Sweeteners
    Newsletter* (USDA),
    10
Sugarholics. *See* Sugar
    addiction.
Sugar-sensitivity, 9
Sulfites, 129
Supplements, dietary,
    179–180
Sweet 'N Low. *See*
    Saccharin.

Takaahushi, Dr. Eyi,
    118
Tannic acid, 118
Tartrazine, 129
Thyroxin, 65
Tooth decay, 97–100
Trace minerals, 25
Truss, Dr. C. Orion,
    96
*Tufts University Diet and
    Nutrition Letter*,
    117
Tyramine, 76

Ulcerative colitis. *See*
    Inflammatory bowel
    disease.
Ulett, Dr. George, 36, 112
Ultraviolet rays, 159
United States Depart-
    ment of Agriculture
    (USDA), 10, 92

Vegetable Chowder, 185
Vegetable recipes,
    188–191

Vegetable Rice Salad, 195
Vegetarian Stew, 191

Walberg, Dr. Otto, 78
Wallach, Dr. Joel, 36, 37,
    104–105
Weight gain, controlling,
    91–94
Wurtman, Dr. Richard,
    132

Zinc, 16, 21, 27, 114